LET MEDITATION MEND YOU

Harness the power of the mind to achieve inner peace

Second Edition

DRs. ESTELLA & JACINTA CK

DocUmeant *Publishing*
244 5th Avenue
Suite G-200
NY, NY 10001
646-233-4366
www.DocUmeantPublishing.com

LET MEDITATION MEND YOU
Second Edition

Published by

DocUmeant Publishing
244 5th Avenue, Suite G-200
NY, NY 10001

646-233-4366

Limit of Liability and Disclaimer of Warranty: The publisher has used its best efforts in preparing this book, and the information provided herein is provided "as is.

Medical Liability Disclaimer: This book is sold with the understanding that the publisher and the author are not engaged in rendering any legal, medical or any other professional services. If expert assistance is required, the services of a competent professional should be sought.

Scripture references marked" KJV" are taken from the King James Version of the Bible.

Scripture quotations marked "NASB" are taken from the New American Standard Bible, Copyright 1960, 1962, 1963, 1971, 1972, 1973, 1975, 1977, 1995 by The Lockman Foundation. Used by permission.

Scripture quotations marked "TNSRB" are taken from The New Scofield Reference Bible, King James Version (New York: Oxford University Press, 1967). The New Scofield Reference Bible contains introductions, annotations, subject chain references, and some word changes in the King James Version that will help the reader.

Editor: Daniel H. Russell, alwaysrussellnessallthetime@yahoo.com

Cover Design by: Patti Knoles, www.virtualgraphicartsdepartment.com

Layout & Design by: DocUmeant Designs, www.DocUmeantDesings.com

Library of Congress Control Number: 2019945158

ISBN13: 978-1-950075-07-2

Dedication

TO MY MOM AND DAD, words cannot express all that you are to me. If not for them, my family and I would not be where we are today. The guidance and love for God they instilled in us is unwavering. They taught me how to love, live, and forgive. I know they are with me in spirit, as I work to share meditation as a means to peace on this earth and preparedness for the eternal one.

Dr. Estella Chavous

Contents

DEDICATION III

ACKNOWLEDGMENTS IX

FOREWORD XI

INTRODUCTION XIII

EDITORS' NOTE XV

CHAPTER 1: HISTORY OF MEDITATION 1

CHAPTER 2: CONCEPTIONS AND MISCONCEPTIONS ABOUT MEDITATION 3

CHAPTER 3: THE BENEFITS OF MEDITATION 7

CHAPTER 4: TYPES OF MEDITATION AND THEIR BENEFITS 11

    Contemplative Centering Prayer Experience 12

    Guided Meditation Experience. 14

    Mindfulness Meditation Experience 16

    Christian Prayer Meditation Experience 18

    Transcendental Meditation Experience. 20

CHAPTER 5: MEDITATION BENEFITS FOR WOMEN IN THE WORKFORCE 23

    Women in the Workplace 24

    Working Women in Leadership 25

    Women's Stress Coping Techniques 27

Stress Therapy and Treatment 28

Science of Meditation .29

Benefits of Meditation for Women 29

CHAPTER 6: MEDITATION AND MUSIC BENEFITS 31

The Science of Music. 31

Music Treatments 33

Benefits of Music. 34

CHAPTER 7: HOW DO I MEDITATE? .37

Learning to Avoid Distractions. 38

Dealing with a Stressful Episode 40

Environmental Concerns. 41

Meditative Techniques 42

Summary. 43

CHAPTER 8: REAL LIFE MEDITATION STORIES. 45

Juliana's Bullying Story 46

Kari's Job Loss Story 48

Candice's Moving Story 50

Tony's Cancer Story 52

Ria's Self-image and Being a Teen Story 54

Jennifer's Student Stress Story 55

Keith and Susan's Divorce Story 57

Colin's Workforce/Work-Life Balance Story 59

Michelle's Death in the Family Story 61

Taryn's Weight-loss Story 63

Kara's Dating Story 64

CHAPTER 9: GROUNDING YOURSELF FOR A SUCCESSFUL MEDITATIVE PRACTICE 67

Learning to Ground Yourself for Success. 67

Get acclimated to your environment 68

Realize your vision. .68

Open your mental capacity 68

Use your inner strength to make change 69

Notice the small and big wins and what prevents your vision 69

Dedicate yourself for effective and continual change 69

CHAPTER 10: THE *LET MEDITATION MEND YOU* GROUNDING GUIDE. 71

Putting the Grounding Guide Into Practice 71

CONTINUED RESEARCH. 79

REFERENCES 81

ABOUT THE AUTHORS. 91

You're looking at a woman 92

I am 93

Acknowledgments

FIRST AND FOREMOST, we want to thank our Lord and Savior Jesus Christ for He is the one that has given us eternal life. He has also given us the ability to love and be accepting of everyone, even those that share different beliefs, for we know that no matter what "his will be done".

To my siblings, aunts, uncles (Rose, Edwin, and Kevin), my son-in-law, husband (Julius), grandchildren, children (Natalia, Isabella, and Nickolas), inspiring us along the way.

To my co-author, business partner, and daughter Jacinta, who is my rock, best friend, and the best child a mother could have.

To my mom, words cannot express all that you are to me.

To our editor Daniel Russell, who not only supported us though the grueling dissertation process, but also has now been commissioned to help us with our laundry list of novels.

To our readers and others who touch our lives every day, thank you. This book would not be possible without you and your support.

Foreword

MANY PEOPLE AVOID MEDITATION because they associate it with a particular religion or faith. If a person belongs to a different religion or is not religious at all, he or she may shy away from meditation due to not wanting to be labeled with that particular faith. However, in 21st century Western culture and practice meditation is so linked to the sciences of mental and emotional health and wellness, stress relief, and positive brain chemistry changes that it often gets completely severed from its religious connections.

Nevertheless, individuals and groups from all religions can still use meditation as an integral part of practicing their particular faith. Accordingly, *Let Meditation Mend You,* which is based on Dr. Estella Chavous' dissertation titled *Effects of Meditation Treatments in Managing Workforce Stress with Women in Leadership,* was written to encourage you to think about meditation in terms of its health benefits as an important part of your daily stress management routine and to eliminate the idea that only people of certain faiths can practice meditation.

This book provides simple overviews of the theory and practice of several common meditation types to ensure that each person makes informed choices on their meditation practices based on sound research and desired outcomes. In short, *Let Meditation Mend You* means that you get to design your own meditation routine to make it take on whatever significance you want it to have in your life, be it health and wellness, faith-based, both, or otherwise.

Introduction

LET MEDITATION MEND YOU will share the history, origin, and benefits of the common forms of meditation. It will provide an introduction to meditation, revealing its overarching healing properties. This book also has a special chapter dedicated to women in the workforce and the effects meditation will have in their roles as future global transformational leaders.

In order to be informed about the art form, it is important that each reader understands its past and present practices. This book is not intended to state findings as facts nor to give readers all they need to know about meditation; it is to give each reader an introduction to the existing research and current practices, enabling you to select the meditation form that works best for you.

Inside *Let Meditation Mend You,* you'll find an overview of the most common forms of meditation and how to practice them should you desire to.

Editors' Note

LET MEDITATION MEND YOU consists of both extensive research into meditation as well as plenty of practical applications and personal stories. As a result, Chapters 5 and 6 of this book contain scientific and medical jargon. This is necessary to establish the credibility of the authors' extensive research into meditation. The authors are not merely presenting their own opinions about meditation; they have thoroughly investigated much literature on the topic.

As is standard with all academic writing in the social sciences, in-text citations and references are by and large written according to APA format. Readers who are interested in this level of extensive research will thoroughly enjoy the scientific and medical jargon found in Chapters 5 and 6. However, if you are not interested in this kind of jargon, please do not pass on *Let Meditation Mend You* until you read the practical applications in Chapter 7, the powerful, personal stories of meditation in Chapter 8, and the authors' personal model of meditation in Chapters 9 and 10.

CHAPTER 1

History of Meditation

SIMILAR TO THE VARYING BELIEFS on the origin of humankind, the practices of meditation span the spectrum in its mental representation. Even the definition of meditation has evolved to incorporate approaches that train the mind comparable to an athlete's training. Regardless of anyone's thoughts on the practice, it has continued to produce therapeutic benefits even through centuries of change and opinions.

But what is the origin of the practice? The answer is that there are many origins and forms of meditation, most of which started with religious, spiritual, or cultural roots. The origins of meditation date back to ancient times, and some have said that primitive humankind even used meditative states while looking into flames of fire. As early as 500 B.C., Buddha represented the art of meditation that spread throughout Asia (Buddhist art, Wikipedia). The opening lines of the *Dhammapada* were spoken by Gotama Buddha 2,500 years ago, illustrating the central theme of Buddhist teaching, the human mind.

Therefore, Buddhism is a series of mental exercises or meditations designed to uncover and cure our psychic aberrations (Burns, 1994).

Other countries also adopted forms of meditation based on the Hindu-based Eastern style. Hindu meditation is defined as a relaxed, contemplative moment where the reflection is on the present. During this reflective moment, the mind is free of all thought, which opens oneself up to spiritual enlightenment and the transformation of attitudes. Your strength is found as you enter deep into your being. This strength is believed to sustain the meditator throughout the day, preventing the calm center from being disturbed. Fear, doubt, and other earthly troubles cannot touch the practitioner of Hindu meditation who has tapped into this strength (Johnson, 2007).

Ancient Jews also practiced meditation. The Old Testament of the Bible references meditation in many of its chapters. As one example, Joshua, who succeeded Moses as God's chosen leader, spoke on the teaching of God in Joshua 1 *"The book of the law shall not depart out of thy mouth, but thou shalt meditate therein day and night, that thou may observe to do according to all that is written"* (v. 8 KJV).

As these examples illustrate, meditation has thousands of years of history and is largely rooted in religion and spirituality. However, despite its ancient roots in these areas, its evolution into a science designed to explore its health advantages should invite all comers to participate in its benefits, whether for religious reasons or otherwise. The body of research on meditation has found it to have positive mental and physical benefits, linking it to better overall health and an improved quality of life. No matter what form of meditation is chosen, its positive benefits have been attested throughout all practices in numerous cultures and religions.

CHAPTER 2

Conceptions and Misconceptions about Meditation

"Meditate . . . some answers can't be found on the Internet." —Julius Kambach

THROUGHOUT THE HISTORY OF HUMAN-KIND, many have felt that the true experience of life comes from listening and being, which many have experienced through meditation. There are many perspectives on meditation that have influenced belief systems and define what it is or isn't. Research with individuals on the subject of meditation uncovered that there are a wide variety of perspectives on the experience or lack of as well as a wide variety of environmental conditions that prevented or encouraged the practice. For those who didn't practice meditation, the four biggest barriers to entry were (1) time, (2) complexity, (3) belief structure, and (4) personality type.

Common comments that prevented individuals from experiencing meditation were:

"Meditation takes too much time that I don't have time for."

|||||||||||||||||||||||||||||||||||||||||||||||||||||||||||||||||||||||||

"Meditation is a complicated laundry list of instructions on breathing, posture, and states of mind."

|||||||||||||||||||||||||||||||||||||||||||||||||||||||||||||||||||||||||

"Meditation is not of my faith or belief structure."

|||||||||||||||||||||||||||||||||||||||||||||||||||||||||||||||||||||||||

"Meditation is too difficult for me because my 'A' personality wouldn't allow me to do it right."

|||||||||||||||||||||||||||||||||||||||||||||||||||||||||||||||||||||||||

On the other hand, those who tried meditation had comments that were tremendously different. Their experiences led them to increases in (1) health, (2) self-awareness/self-reflection, (3) faith, and (4) purpose. Common comments from their experiences were:

"Meditation has saved my life and improved my overall health."

|||||||||||||||||||||||||||||||||||||||||||||||||||||||||||||||||||||||||

"Meditation has helped me with self-awareness and self-reflection."

|||||||||||||||||||||||||||||||||||||||||||||||||||||||||||||||||||||||||

"Meditation has brought me closer to my faith and my purpose in this world."

|||||||||||||||||||||||||||||||||||||||||||||||||||||||||||||||||||||||||

The results from these findings further support potential misconceptions about meditation and the need to fill gaps of understanding in respect to this practice.

Numerous scholarly studies have found that meditation supports stress release and anxiety release, improves mental and physical health, decreases fatigue and insomnia, and provides an environment of peacefulness and calm. Meditation is not new; it has been a documented practice for thousands of years. But even with the research, testimonials, and miracles seen in its practice, there are still limits to its use due to misconceptions and lack of knowledge.

Some of the more common beliefs about meditation are that it is difficult to learn, is time consuming, takes years to master, creates a hypnotic state, and is rooted in culture and religious doctrines. In my recent research, I examined women in leadership and how meditation could help them in their leadership roles. In that study, it was found that ten minutes a day was more beneficial than an hour of meditation. This was just one population, but similar research on other populations has yielded similar results, suggesting that extended time is not a factor in the benefits seen. Additionally, the population chosen varied in the length of time they practiced, and numerous forms of meditation were represented in the study. This suggests that the time to learn the practice was more a consequence of discipline and commitment to the practice versus any skill needed.

Another conception about meditation is that only people of certain faiths or religions can practice it. The history of meditation is in fact rooted in culture and religion, but one must remember that the use of meditation can be found in many religions, even to the extent that it is part of their doctrine and teaching. Also, as with many alternative practices movements, its spread into Western culture has caused an evolution in meditative practice—its current use in Western culture is so far removed from its cultural and religious roots that it is often not affiliated at all with religion. In fact, the practice of meditation has become a brain science, as its benefits have shown to result in chemical and structural changes in the brain and body with regular use.

A question that has raised concerns is if meditation creates a hypnotic state for those interested in the practice and if one still remains in control of the brain during the practice. According to the American Society of Clinical Hypnosis (ASCH), hypnosis is a state of inner absorption, concentration, and focused attention enabling us to use our minds more powerfully. So this definition would support meditation being a hypnotic state but one we voluntarily put ourselves in when we focus on anything. But is this state mind control?

A researcher named De Vol (1974) performed an interesting study that may unlock the answer. He studied Buddhist monks who meditated and Pentecostal Christians who used *glossolalia* prayer (a prayer in tongues which involves music, scripture reading, prayer, and meditation) to see if each group was still in control of their brains during both practices. While comparing the two, he found that the Buddhist monks still remained in control of the brains, but the Pentecostal glossolalia prayer group had an altered state of consciousness and lost control of their brains during the process.

This study suggests that in meditative states individuals are in control of their minds, unlike what appeared to happen in glossolalia prayer that renders a person in an altered state of consciousness. This finding could open up a new area of research for brain science, meditation, and glossolalia prayer.

CHAPTER 3

The Benefits of Meditation

"Active meditation exemplifies the life you long to live." —Paul Hines

THE SCIENCE OF MEDITATION yields a number of health benefits ranging from enhanced memory power to increased creativity and stress reduction. Paul Hines, an accomplished musician and friend of mine, said, "Active meditation exemplifies the life you long to live" (personal communication). Although his belief on meditation is similar to others' in its ability to produce beneficial results, the practice and selection process can be complicated. Not only are there misunderstandings about the practice, but also the different types of meditation make selecting a form complicated.

Despite these complexities, countless reasons support the practice of meditation, the foremost of these reasons being its many documented benefits.

Most would agree that there is an overarching need for medicine to be more preventative than reactive, to replace bandages with cures and prevention. Because of this, the field of preventative and integrative medicine is growing. The research in preventative medicine has revealed that the root of most diseases is inflammation and stress, both of which can be managed.

Inflammation by definition is a response to cellular injury that is marked by capillary dilatation, leukocytic infiltration, redness, heat, and pain that serves as a mechanism initiating the elimination of noxious agents and damaged tissue (Inflammation definition, Webster Dictionary). Chronic inflammation has been seen in asthma, peptic ulcers, tuberculosis, rheumatoid arthritis, chronic periodontitis, ulcerative colitis, chronic sinusitis, chronic active hepatitis, Alzheimer's, anemia, stroke, congestive heart and kidney failure, and more. The fact that the human immune system drives the inflammatory process in disease is well established. Common therapies suppress it but rarely work to use alternative therapies that turn off the response causing the inflammation.

Stress also plays a venomous role in disease. There is good and bad stress, each beginning with stressors. Acute stress, commonly called good stress, is brief in duration and has proven to be beneficial in creating motivation. Chronic stress, or bad stress, is more severe than good stress and has been associated with psychosis and physiological damage. Stress has been defined as a constellation of events consisting of a stressor that precipitates a reaction in the brain that in turn activates physiological fight-or-flight systems in the body (Firdaus, William, Eric, & Bruce, 2012, p. 1346).

Psychological stress results in a rise in cortisol level, influencing psychological and physiological parameters and health outcomes in health and disease (Fan, Tang, & Posner, 2014, p. 222). Stress causes increases in cortisol along with a host of inflammation triggers like diet, infections, and hormonal metabolic and neurological changes that break down in the gut.

Previous work has shown that mind-body therapies offer many psychological and health functioning benefits, including reduction in disease symptoms, improvements in coping with stress, behavior regulation, and improvements in quality of life and well-being (Morgan, Irwin, Chung, & Wang, 2014, p. 1). One study found that the decreased expression of pro-inflammatory genes (*RIPK2* and *COX2*) might represent some of the mechanisms underlying the therapeutic potential of mindfulness-based interventions (Kaliman et al., 2014). Meditation has also been shown to boost the human immune system. A recent study uncovered that mind-body therapies were positively associated with decreased C- reactive protein and other cellular inflammation marker levels in patients with type 2 diabetes, cancer, or heart failure, and also in the elderly with depression and cardiovascular disease risk factors (Kaliman et al., 2014, p. 9).

Furthermore, a 2011 MIT study found that people who were trained to meditate over an eight week period were better able to control a specific type of brain waves called alpha rhythms, which minimize distractions. This result indicates that meditation might be effective for pain relief. In the study, subjects trained themselves to focus on physical sensations from certain parts of their bodies, leading researchers to believe that people who suffer from chronic conditions could be able to train themselves to "turn down the volume" (Kerr, Sacchet, Lazar, Moore, & Jones, 2013, p. 32) on pain.

As further benefits of meditation, Teper and Inzlicht (2013) found that meditation is related to better executive control and improves executive functioning, resulting in increased acceptance of emotional states (p. 8). Additionally, Ding, Tang, Tang, and Posner (2014) discovered that creativity performance through divergent thinking tasks is improved with meditation (p. 5). Moreover, McCreary and Alderson (2013) found that participants who practiced meditation ultimately experienced increased harmony in their relationships on a day-to-day basis through improving their self-control and communication and increasing their openness (p. 109). This body of research has resulted in the National Center for Complementary and Alternative Medicine designating mind-body therapies as a top research priority (Morgan, Irwin, Chung, & Wang, 2014, p. 1).

Although alternative interventions like meditation have shown promise and have resulted in positive outcomes, their effects are somewhat inconsistent, as are their varying techniques, styles, and origins. The problems in this field lie in the study of visualization and its effectiveness. The idea that the mind may influence the body has long been intriguing. Because of this new emergence in meditation utilization, alternative interventions are now a focus in research and in mainstream holistic practices.

CHAPTER 4

Types of Meditation and their Benefits

"This class is making me use my intelligence."
—Isabella Kambach (age 6)

MY DAUGHTER, WHO IS SIX YEARS OLD, started her first day of first grade in September, 2015. When I asked her how her first day went, she replied, "This class is making me use my intelligence." This quote by my six-year-old daughter is so fitting for this chapter because understanding the types and benefits of meditation can do just that . . . expand your intelligence. This chapter provides an overview of the main types and the benefits they offer.

There are several types of meditation that are differentiated by being new, traditional, and individualized. Additionally, the length of time of meditation has been questioned. Research focused on state versus trait changes in short-term and long-term meditations indicates an immediate increase in concentration abilities with shorter-term meditation practice. However, sustaining longer-term state changes requires on-going practice (Romano, 2014, p. 9).

If you research meditation, there are a host of options to choose from, even some that are specifically created to reflect one's individual beliefs. It is important that you align yourself with the type of meditation that speaks to you so that you are relaxed. Once you find the meditation that is right for you, you can go into your meditative state no matter the situation or environment you're faced with.

It is important to remember that meditation is personal and should reflect you and your foundation. In the following pages, you will be presented with the most common types of meditation. Keep in mind that there are many forms to choose from as well as more information to be read on each type. Because of this, one's research or experience should not be limited to just the ones in this book, as it is important that you find a style and practice that is right for you. The ones selected in this book were chosen because of the large body of research on their origins, goals, practices, and benefits and their being commonly practiced in mainstream society.

CONTEMPLATIVE CENTERING PRAYER EXPERIENCE

"The Trust for the Meditation Process embodies and promotes deep insight into the contemporary direction of social change. Its support of groups which give guidance into spiritual experience, not just spiritual talk, makes it a leader in its field." —Laurence Freeman OSB

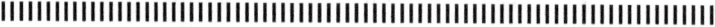

||||||||||||||||||||||||||||||||||||||||||||||||||||||||||||||||||||||||||||

Meditation Type: Contemplative Centering Prayer

Origin: Contemplative centering prayer has a long Christian history and has representation in every age. A form of contemplative prayer was first practiced and taught by the Desert Fathers of Egypt, Palestine, and Syria, including Evagrius, St. Augustine, and St. Gregory the Great in the West and Pseudo-Dionysius and the Hesychasts in the East (contemplative Outreach). In the first 16 centuries of the Christian era, St. Gregory the Great summed up contemplative prayer as the knowledge of God that combined the word in the scripture and a gift from God.

In the 20th and 21st centuries, initiatives were taken by various religious orders, notably by the Jesuits and Discalced Carmelites, to renew the contemplative orientation of their founders and to share their spirituality with laypeople. The result was centering prayer based on the wisdom teaching of Jesus in the Sermon on the Mount:

> "... When you pray, go to your inner room, close the door and pray to your Father in secret. And your Father, who sees in secret, will repay you" (Matthew 6:6 NASB).

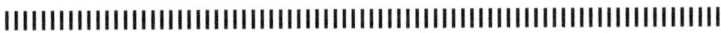

|||||||||||||||||||||||||||||||||||||||||||||||||||||||||||||||||||||||||||||||||||||||||||||||||

Goal: Contemplative centering prayer belief is that oneness with God is a gift that cannot be achieved at will. It is a total transformation by giving one's whole being to God. The result is a divine union and relationship to God. Contemplative centering prayer meditation has evolved and is based on Thomas Keating's teachings in which this form of meditation attempts to provide a method to respond to God's initiative and gives a means to be present to God. Mindfulness, when used in centering prayer, is "knowing what you are doing while you are doing it" (Wilhoit, 2014, p. 109). Contemplative centering prayer operates in grace where one cooperates with the gift of God's presence.

Practice: Contemplative centering prayer occurs while sitting in silence for an established period of time with the intention of being present before God. One meditates on a sacred word. Catholic nuns provide evidence in support of the role of contemplative prayer and meditation in generating the joy and serenity that Jesus' allusion to the hidden treasure in Matthew 13:44 envisions.

Benefits: *Re-sculpture of the brain:* Contemplative centering prayer meditation has been shown to literally "re-sculpt" our brains over time through contemplative spiritual practice and mindfulness meditation, helping us embrace the treasures of love, peace, and serenity even in these anxious times (Wilhoit, 2014, p. 113).

- *Life Skill of Mindfulness:* Contemplative centering prayer promotes the life skill of mindfulness. Mindfulness when used in centering prayer is "knowing what you are doing while you are doing it" (Wilhoit, 2014, p. 113). Although the word mindful is used a few times in English translations of the Bible (ten times in the KJV), the term could easily be substituted with a synonym like "attentive". The construct of mindfulness per se is not central in Keating's teachings (Wilhoit, 2014, p. 114). However, he advocated contemplative centering prayer as a way of growing into a state of equanimity where one is less captivated by the opinions of others and is more able to hear from God.

- Ultimate Union with God: A divine union and relationship to God is created.

GUIDED MEDITATION EXPERIENCE

"Guided meditation is a voice inspired by your guide that opens you to love, truth, and a path toward revelations." —**Estella Chavous**

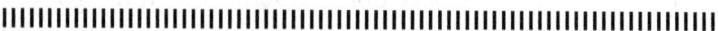

||||||||||||||||||||||||||||||||||||||||||||||||||||||||||||||||||||||||||||||||

Meditation Type: Guided Meditation

Origin: Guided meditation is another form of meditation that is becoming popular in various populations. Its origins can be found in contemplative, Christian, Buddhist, and other traditions. In the 12th century, the Buddhist monks developed steps to meditation, which are read, ponder, pray, and contemplate—tenets that are similar across all practices (History of Meditation, April, 2012). Others can find guidance in your group, your guide, or intuitive guidance from within.

Goal: The goals of guided meditation are to clear the mind to facilitate relaxation, to reduce stress, and to enhance personal and spiritual growth. The spiritual aspect does not have to be emphasized for those who do not adhere to a particular faith; many use guided meditation with a focus on improved health. A guide can use many techniques to induce the mind to a state of calm and thereby reduce stress. Some forms work to fill the mind with positive imagery, affirmations, etc.

Practice: Guided meditation is often practiced with a recorded or in-person guide. As the sessions continue, the need for a guide decreases. The auditory guidance points out imagery, imagines affirmations, and states peacefulness or imagined desired experiences. Through these guided states of consciousness, focus is on one's awareness and attention. A lot of concentration is focused on breathing and verbal instructions teaching one to relax and clear the mind.

Benefits: *Intervention and Health*—Guided meditation has been commonly used in intervention, and health benefits have been reported (Bedford, 2012, p. 25).

- *Combats Illness*—It has been shown to lower hypertension, reducing the onset of asthma, allergies, and pain.
- *Increases relaxation*—creates a sense of balance; reduces depression, anxiety, and stress; and increases coping skills.

MINDFULNESS MEDITATION EXPERIENCE

"Happiness does not depend on what you have or who you are. It solely relies on what you think." —Buddha

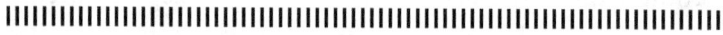

|||||||||||||||||||||||||||||||||||||||||||||||||||||||||||||||||||||||||||||||

Meditation Type: Mindfulness Meditation

Origin: The origin of mindfulness meditation is derived from ancient Buddhist and yoga practices. It is a mental state characterized by nonjudgmental awareness, teaching people to live each moment as it unfolds. It is a state of rigidity in which one adheres to a single perspective and acts automatically. When one is mindful, one is trapped in a rigid mindset and is oblivious to context or perspective. Practitioners have adopted variations of this form of meditation specific to stress reduction. These nonreligious programs are anchored in the development of awareness in moment-to-moment experience.

Goal: The goal involves focusing attention on the present circumstances and accepting them without judgment (Tanner et al., 2009, p. 575). Practitioners learn to be mindful and calm their minds.

Practice: This practice is an accepting and non-judgmental focus of one's attention on emotions, thoughts, and sensations. The focus is on an object (like breathing). Mindfulness means paying attention in a particular way: on purpose, in the present moment, and non-judgmentally. Mindfulness represents a method of learning to relate directly to whatever is happening in one's life, a way of taking charge of one's life, a way of doing something for yourself that no one else can do for you-consciously and systematically working with your own stress, pain, illness, and the challenges and demands of everyday life.

Benefits: Research has correlated meditation with changes in brain chemistry. A recent study led by Massachusetts General Hospital researchers and senior author Dr. Sara Lazar has documented structural changes in the brains of individuals who participated in mindfulness-based stress reduction. Lazar found that practicing mindfulness meditation thickens the brain's mid-prefrontal cortex mid-insular region, "This study demonstrates that changes in brain structure may underlie some of these [cognitive and psychological] improvements and that people are not just feeling better because they are spending time relaxing" (Hölzel et al., 2011, p. 537).

For over 30 years, researchers Langer and Kabat-Zinn have each worked independently in the mindfulness area with limited contact between them (Hart, Ivtzan, & Hart, 2013, p.461). Research has shown that Langer's model seems to capture the cognitive attributes that underlie creativity. The model (a) is more Western and scientific in nature, (b) targets healthy people in everyday settings, and (c) requires brief instructional, short-lived interventions (Hart, Ivtzan, & Hart, 2013, p. 461). Kabat-Zinn's multifaceted construct seems to accentuate the metacognitive processes and the accommodating stance involved in mindfulness. It more closely mirrors Buddhist religious practices, is used more in clinical settings, and offers therapeutic packages (Hart, Ivtzan, & Hart, 2013, p. 461). Both models have proven to help elevate positive psychological mind states, to mitigate physical disorders, and to improve aspects of well-being in both healthy and clinical patients. It has been successful in alleviating pain, depression, anxiety, and stress as well as in helping with coping skills.

CHRISTIAN PRAYER MEDITATION EXPERIENCE

> *"This book of the law shall not depart out of thy mouth, but thou shalt meditate therein day and night, that thou mayest observe to do according to all that is written therein: for then thou shalt make thy way prosperous, and then thou shalt have good success."* —Joshua 1:8

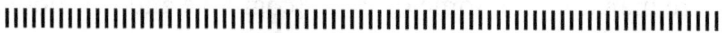

||||||||||||||||||||||||||||||||||||||||||||||||||||||||||||||||||||||||||||||||||||||

Meditation Type: Christian Prayer Meditation Experience

Origin: In the beginning God created the heavens and earth. Now the earth was without form and void and darkness was upon the face of the deep. And the Spirit of God moved upon the face of the waters and it was changed by a simple voice *"Let there be Light"* (Genesis 1:1-3a, TNSRB).

Christians often avoid meditation because they associate it with Eastern religions. However, the Christian Bible is filled with examples of meditation. For Christians, the Old Testament of the Bible is the preparation for Christ. In the Gospels he manifested to the world, in the Acts he is preached and his gospel is propagated in the world, in the Epistles his gospel is explained, and in Revelation all the purposes of God in and through Christ are consummated. In the Old Testament there are two primary Hebrew words for meditation: *Haga* (הגה), which means to utter, groan, meditate, or ponder, and *Sihach* (חיש), which means to muse, rehearse in one's mind, or contemplate. These words can also be translated as dwell, diligently consider, and heed.

Goal: In the Bible, which is the word of God for Christians, the word "meditate" or the act of meditation is mentioned 20 times. Piper (1999) wrote that the word of God inspires, informs, and incarnates. The word inspires Christians, meaning that the word commands

Christians to pray, makes promises to Christians of what God will do if they pray, and tells stories of great men and women of prayer. The word informs, meaning it tells Christians what to pray and itself becomes the content of prayer, and the word incarnates Christians, meaning that prayers are often invisible and concealed in the soul and in the closet and in the church. Our thoughts determine our behavior, so what we think about is very important. That is why Christians believe God wants them to think about his word, which is the same thing as meditating on it. Meditation is *focused* thinking, so for Christians, the goal of meditative prayer is to focus on God's word so it can transform them to what God wants them to be.

Practice: The definition of meditation is to engage in contemplation or reflection. With Christian prayer it is a concentrated focus upon God's word to increase awareness on him and what he would have Christians to do. To pray means to speak to God with adoration, confession, supplication, intercession, or thanksgiving. The practice of meditation in the Christian form can be done with a guide who can lead you in biblical principles or in the word or through silent contemplation on a sacred word, affirmation or scripture—all of which are done by turning the mind over to God and his word.

Benefit: One of God's goals for Christians is to build a relationship with Jesus Christ and to fill their minds with Christ's word so that Christians can help others (through acts of benevolence like feeding the poor, helping the homeless, visiting the incarcerated, etc.) and themselves (through gaining control of greed, anger, adulterous desires, etc.). In addition, James 5:16 says, *"The effective prayer of a righteous person can accomplish much".* The benefits are all encompassing and can be seen in miracles in mental, physical, and spiritual health as well as in inner peace, self-growth, faith, and awareness gained.

TRANSCENDENTAL MEDITATION EXPERIENCE

"The thing about Meditation is: You become more and more you." —David Lynch

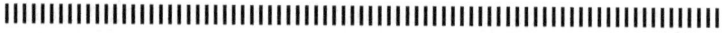

||||||||||||||||||||||||||||||||||||||||||||||||||||||||||||||||||||||||||

Meditation Type: Transcendental Meditation

Origin: Hinduism concentrative (transcendental) meditation includes the categories of open awareness, guided practice, and mindfulness meditation. It had its beginnings in the Far East and then spread to the western world. It is based on Vedic Meditation, which is a simple, natural process that progressively improves the balance of the physical nervous system through regularly alternating profound restfulness with normal daily activity (Mason, 2014). Every physical activity has a corresponding mental activity and every mental activity has a corresponding physical activity, so the body and mind are not two separate things but part of a unified whole which should at all times be working in complete harmony.

Transcendental meditation is a relatively new form of meditating in comparison with Yoga and Buddhist meditation. It was developed by Maharishi Mahesh Yogi in 1957 as a way of developing the mind so that a person can rise above or "transcend" beyond the noise and stress of daily life. Maharishi Mahesh Yogi was a student of the famous Hindu Guru Swami Brahmananda Saraswati (Mason, 2014). Although transcendental meditation does not have any religious affiliation, it did have a political association in the Natural Law Party. This political party was formed in 1992 with the goal of using the principles of the meditation as a way of finding ways to solve the problems of society—crime, injustice, economics, and environmental issues.

Goal: Transcendental meditation is a simple technique and is not a philosophy. It is natural, simple, and effortless. It is designed to take the mind from active levels of thinking to a state of less mental activity, and its goal is to create inner peace and wellness.

> *"The goal of the Transcendental Meditation technique is the state of enlightenment. This means we experience that inner calmness, that quiet state of least excitation, even when we are dynamically busy."* —Maharishi

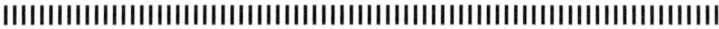

The diagram on the next page summarizes the most common types of meditation. Its purpose is to not only introduce you to the origin, goal, and practice type, but to also help you understand that a universal platform of meditation can be practiced irrespective of your belief system. This illustration has been used along with the G.R.O.U.N.D model as a reference and/or training tool.

Meditation Types

Guided Meditation (GM)

Origin: Diverse
Goal: Clarity, relaxation, stress, and spiritual growth
Practice: Guided state of consciousness through voice or recordings.

Mindfulness Meditation (MM)

Origin: Buddhist
Goal: Clarity, relaxation, stress, & spiritual growth
Practice: Accepting and Non-judgmental focus of ones attention on emotions, thoughts, and sensations (like breathing).

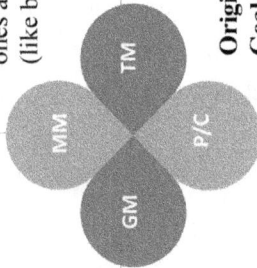

Prayer/Centering

Origin: Christian/Father Keating
Goal: Filling the mind and creating a relationship with Jesus Christ
Practice: Meditation in the strict sense. Meditation of the heart, focusing on a sacred word, affirmation etc.

Transcendental (TM)

Origin: Hinduism
Goal: Inner peace and wellness
Practice: Meditate using sounds or mantra's (sacred utterance) practices 2x per day.

MM   TM   GM   P/C

CHAPTER 5

Meditation Benefits for Women in the Workforce

"I win!" —Nickolas Kambach (age 3)

IN THE WORDS OF MY THREE-YEAR-OLD GRANDSON, when you do meditation, you win! Meditation has been proven to have a huge impact on stress levels for women in the workforce. With the shifting roles of women from traditional to non-traditional roles as well as with the current trend of women in leadership, women have become particularly vulnerable to stress. This stress is causing huge problems with health, which could affect women's economic, family, and social health across the world. This chapter will focus on this special population as an example of the positive impact meditation can have. It will discuss the epidemic of stress, women in the workplace, women in leadership, women's stress coping techniques, stress therapies and treatment, the science of meditation, and the benefits of meditation in this population.

WOMEN IN THE WORKPLACE

Nearly one billion women around the world could enter the global economy during the coming decade. They are poised to play significant roles in countries around the world—as significant as that of the billion-plus populations of India and China (Empowering the third billion, 2012, p. 5). Employers will have different concerns to address with women than they did with men in the workplace due to this change in demographic.

A U.S. Bureau of Labor and Statistics (2012) report showed that the United States women's labor force participation rate peaked at 60% in 1999, following several decades in which women increasingly entered the labor market. In 2006, the proportion of women to men in the workplace was nearly equal at 49% and 51%, respectively (JaekwonKo, Seung,UK, & Smith-Walter, 2013, p .546). In 2011, 58.1% of women were in the labor force (Department of Labor, 2005). Research indicates that working women have unique obstacles that include discrimination, stereotyping, conflicting demands of marriage, and work/life and social isolations, all of which fuel stress-related concerns (Nelson & Quick, 1985, p. 209).

A recent study in India has highlighted the existence of a glass ceiling in industries like IT. In such industries, the women workforce is mostly concentrated at lower levels of the job hierarchy (Nelson & Quick, 1985, p. 179). Another study showed that managers might not promote women because of taste-based or statistical discrimination (Adams & Kirchmaier, 2013, p. 2). Additionally, almost all reports pertaining to the topic have cited the costs of managing work and family as a major barrier (Adams & Kirchmaier, 2013, p. 2). Furthermore, Madan (2013) stated that policy makers should focus more on gender planning and gender sensitive priorities to promote more gender inclusive information. In other words, the policy towards women should shift from equality to equity (Madan, 2013,

p. 177). The above stress related concerns could greatly affect organizations' output and growth as a result of this changing demographic. Decreased productivity, litigation, absenteeism, poor health, and work-life conflict could result if these issues are not addressed.

Studies have found that women often experience work/family conflict, resulting in greater stress and burnout. Women at work are balancing the shift from traditional to non-traditional roles while trying to keep up with work demands. A possible solution is to create more flexibility for women in the workplace to support their unique needs. Research suggests that academics and policy makers seek to understand workplace flexibility and its antecedents and consequences to better predict the work/family interface as well as to inform workplace flexibility policy initiatives (Hill et al., 2008, p. 179).

Gender exclusion in organizations must also be considered. It results in consequences for both men and women and affects health outcomes for everyone (Elwér, Harryson, Bolin, & Hammarström, 2013, p. 1). Gender equality is multidimensional and includes division of labor, emotions, symbolic representation, and power in decision-making. Although women dominate many labor forces, their numbers are not reflective of their power.

WORKING WOMEN IN LEADERSHIP

Women are beginning to take more leadership positions within corporations. However, despite the increase in numbers, research has amply demonstrated that accomplished, high-potential women who are evaluated as competent managers often fail the likability test. Conversely, competence and likability tend to go hand in hand for similarly accomplished men. Richardson (2010) concluded that men and women are generally treated differently in business. He also deduced that despite women's hard work to gain acceptance, they still face challenges due to gender.

Another study found that entry into the workplace is associated with stronger links between financial strain, parenting stress, and depressive effects in women (Gyamfi, Brooks-Gunn, & Jackson, 2001, p. 1). This becomes a greater problem when examining gender diversity, especially in executive-level positions. Studies illustrate that women in senior executive, manager, or other supervisory positions frequently encounter unclear promotion opportunities, concerns that home might interfere with work quality, and apprehension from the potential impossibility of reconciling others' conflicting demands (Rogers & Li, 1994, p. 599). In addition, common stressors such as glass-ceiling barriers, differences in gender socialization, work-related discrimination, and gender-role stereotyping often occur.

Women entrepreneurs represent a population of business owners experiencing a large surge in its growth rate. The National Association of Women Business Owners declared 2013 as the "year of the female entrepreneur", which stemmed from women entrepreneurs' emergence as the fastest growing sector of small businesses all over the world. Additionally, the Women-Owned Businesses Report, commissioned by American Express, discovered the presence of more than 8.6 million women-owned businesses in the U.S.—an increase of 59% since 1997. These businesses employ 7.8 million people and generate more than $1.3 trillion in revenue (McMahon, 2013, p. 29).

Women's entry into entrepreneurship has resulted in increased stress with founding companies' leaders. A recent article expressed that nine out of ten startup company founders experience stress linked to factors caused by worrying about funding, taxes, and payroll obligations. To mitigate these stress triggers, founders like Russell D'Souza of SeatGeek, Daniel Robichaud of PasswordBox, and Daniella Yacobovsky of BaubleBar have advocated the following five tips: knowing when to take a break, appreciating your family, thinking strategically, feeding your favorites, and embracing insanity (Stepoe, Andrew & Mika Kivimaki, 2013 p. 34).

Finding ways to accurately measure the cost of stress or to institute treatment programs that maintain sustainable levels of stress reduction within workplaces can be problematic. Stress management programs are a common element in health promotion and employee wellness programs. The challenge becomes finding detailed, written descriptions of the implementation and delivery methods of stress management programs to further develop evidence based stress reduction interventions that are specific to worksites and are founded on prior evidence based outcomes (Werneburg et al., 2011, p. 357). Vanithamani and Menon (2012) analyzed women business entrepreneurs to discover whether or not having facilitative leadership through group membership empowered women to change. The self-maintained nature of these findings notwithstanding, the results demonstrated positive outcomes when women entrepreneurs belonged to groups.

WOMEN'S STRESS COPING TECHNIQUES

Organizations are beginning to progress in the ways in which they are helping women deal with stress related issues. Competition for survival, performances for excellence, and complexities of work design have contributed to enormous work-life stress among employees, leading to depression and anxiety. Mentoring, coaching, counseling, and employee assistance program initiatives help facilitate employee well-being (Nair & Xavier, 2012, p. 67).

A widespread notion in the coping literature assumes that coping strategies are independent and that individuals are prone to use one type over another (Eisenbarth, 2012, p. 142). Research has revealed that coping strategies range from problem focus (looking to elevate the problem), emotional focus (alleviating discomfort by altering perception), or engagement focus (aiming at dealing with stressors or related emotions). But research has also illustrated that the effectiveness of each strategy is not mutually exclusive and does not work with each other separately (Nielsen & Knardahl, 2014, p. 148).

An important implication for practice, cluster analytic techniques can assist health professionals in identifying distinct coping profiles to which individuals may belong. These techniques can subsequently shape intervention designs to the unique dispositions and risks of the targeted group, preventing the use of dysfunctional coping strategies related to poor or good mental health (Eisenbarth, 2012, p. 149).

STRESS THERAPY AND TREATMENT

The brain controls how humans react to stress. Environmental stimuli that influence social and emotional behavior constantly influence the brain. Studies in both animals and in humans provide a foundation that supports evidence suggesting that interventions ranging from moderate physical exercise to cognitive therapy induce plasticity-related alteration of the brain and support a range of positive behavior outcomes (McEwen, 2013, p. 1). Social and emotional behavior is adapted by experience, and evidence indicates that stress can produce modifications in behavior. Recent interventions such as meditation and cognitive therapy can enhance self-control and self-regulation. Additionally, mindfulness meditation has been shown to strengthen selective and other aspects of attention and executive function (McEwen, 2013, p. 2).

Grafton, Gillespie, and Henderson (2010) proposed that many people view the development of resilience in individuals and organizations as a potential answer to the stress associated with contemporary lifestyles and workplaces. Studies have shown an evolution of inquiry into resilience, but the most recent wave of research views resilience in terms of innate energy or motivating life forces within people that enable them to cope with adversity, to learn from experience, and to engage in cognitive transformations. This wave of research points to the development of resilience through holistic self-care practices such as mindfulness meditation (p. 700).

SCIENCE OF MEDITATION

Meditation, prayer, yoga, somatic therapies, and biofeedback constitute a vast array of complementary modalities available to behavioral medicine practitioners to manage symptoms of disease and the underlying thoughts, feelings, and emotions that influence health. This multidisciplinary new wave of medicine emphasizes the patient's active role in maintaining health and preventing illness (Davidson & McEwen, 2012, p. 6). Meditation has proven to be beneficial in improving health, the efficacy of executive processing, and attention to detail (Hawkins, 2013, p. 71). Problems, however, arise when attempting to identify the degree to which meditation affects outcomes and when attempting to measure its effectiveness in vulnerable populations. Furthermore, the ability to differentiate and select the appropriate meditation treatment can be formidable.

BENEFITS OF MEDITATION FOR WOMEN

However, despite these potential challenges, various target groups and populations have benefited from the use of meditation. With the influx of women and the stress they experience in the workplace, employers face challenges in alleviating stress for these women. The research presented in this chapter has shown that meditation has proven to be beneficial for reducing numerous medical ailments, including stress. Although more research into alternative treatments needs to be conducted, sufficient evidence suggests that women can benefit from meditation as a way to reduce stress.

This chapter has focused on stress in women in the workforce as well as the benefits of meditation for this population; however, it must be stressed (pun intended) that meditation is for men as well.

Men experience their own stressors in the workforce and in other aspects of their lives, and they too can reap tremendous mental, emotional, and physical health benefits from practicing meditation. *Let Meditation Mend You* is for you, no matter your gender.

CHAPTER 6

Meditation and Music Benefits

"Opening oneself to music and meditation can lead you to an enlightened self and a purpose-filled life." —JacintaCk

THE SCIENCE OF MUSIC

THERE IS LIMITED but intriguing literature on the use of music in organizations, stretching back to the days of the engineering revolution (Styhre, 2013). Music has been long used and thought to have had positive therapeutic properties. Studies that measure music's impact on health and stress reductions are beginning to surface in the literature. But despite these newly emerging investigations, using music treatment for stress reduction remains an unexplored option in many organizations. A recent study investigated the effects of listening to music and demonstrated its effectiveness in reducing stress in women (Lai & Li, 2011), opening the possibility for using music treatments as a strategy in work related settings.

Past research has shown that a balanced brain induces healthier living. Balanced brainwaves help to enhance critical learning (left brain) and creativity (right brain). Therefore, it is assumed that those who use both sides of their brains maximize productivity. A recent study showed that listening to live violin music results in the subject's left and right brain, especially in Alpha band, being more balanced (Hassan, Murat, Ross, Mohd-Zain, & Buniyamin, 2011, p.1).

Will and Berg (2007) found that different brainwave frequencies show synchronies related to different perceptual, motor, or cognitive states. Brainwaves have also been shown to synchronize with external stimuli with repetition rates of ca. 10-40 Hz. Periodic auditory stimulation produces a mixture of evoked and induced, rate-specific and rate-independent increases in stimulus related brainwave synchronization that are likely to affect various cognitive functions. The synchronization responses in the delta range may form part of the neurophysiological processes underlying time coupling between rhythmic sensory input and motor output (Will & Berg, 2007, p. 1).

Csabai (2013) shared another stress intervention, which uses *frequency following response* in brainwave entrainment, aiding in the removal or changing of unwanted behavior patterns and attitudes. Frequency following response can also assist with affirmations and visualization of one's goals. In addition, binaural beats *(brainwave audio)* can be used to achieve different mind states and reach deep relaxation and meditation, and they also greatly influence self-improvement and overall health. Brainwave entrainment occurs when the internal processes within the brain are mirroring an external stimulus, and it is made up of four frequencies. The first frequency, alpha, is normally associated with a relaxed, peaceful state and operates between 8 and 13 cycles per second. It is experienced during daydreaming, fantasizing, and creative visualization. The second, beta, is associated with our normal brain rhythm in a wakeful state, operating between 13 and 40 cycles per second. Beta is experienced when a person is thinking, alert, conscious, and logical. The third, theta, represents the state in which we can access our subconscious and operates between 4 and 8 cycles per second. It is activated during dream sleep and deep music and is the brain state normally associated with creative thinking and allows us to tap into our inner genius. The last frequency is Delta, the lowest frequency, and it operates between 0.5 and 4 cycles per second. Delta frequencies are produced during deep sleep (Csabai, 2013).

MUSIC TREATMENTS

Music therapists have focused on the benefits and pragmatic uses of music but rarely on the healing aspect. Music treatments, also referred to as sound healing, is an alternative healing method that uses new age music, opera, and classical music to soothe (Campbell, 2009). According to Yehuda (2011), there are three therapeutic functions attributed to music—restoring the soul or body, creating the sensation of pleasure through movement, and inducing catharsis that purges the soul of emotional conflict (p. 1). In one research study, the power of music and vibrations showed a positive effect on the human biological system (Clair & Memmott, 2008). Another study highlights the inherent qualities of music and suggests that the integration of music has therapeutic outcomes (Bae, 2012). One study found that the type of music matters. Music with upbeat tempos, such as hip-hop, rap, heavy metal, and pop should be avoided, as they do not support the relaxation response in the body and can increase adrenaline due to their upbeat nature (Campbell & Doman, 2011).

According to Bruscia (1989), group music therapy is the use of music or music activities as a stimulus for promoting new behaviors and exploring pre-determined individual or group goals in a group setting. The four advantages of using music are its ability to evoke feelings, to provide a vehicle for expression, to stimulate verbalizations, and to provide a common starting place. Receptive music therapy bases its assumption on a piece of music that can evoke a specific personal value in individuals (p. 179-80). Lastly, Robb et al. (1995) described music assisted relaxation, which serves to facilitate the images described and experienced during intervention and is used in conjunction with guided imagery and deep breathing exercises.

In a study completed by Dritsas, Platis, and Cokkinons (2000), it was stated that 78% of patients showed a greater than 50% reduction in stress with use of music according to visual analogue scale analysis. But despite these apparently groundbreaking statistics, McDermott, Crellin, Ridder, and Orrell (2013) asserted that the future of music therapy study might need to be re-defined to the realistic and clinically relevant goal for this population on the basis of a clear theoretical framework. The authors also said that more important is the issue of determining the long-term benefits of music therapy and how music therapy relates to stress reduction (McDermott et al., 2013).

BENEFITS OF MUSIC

According to Tseng, Chen, and Lee (2010), using music to tackle both psychological and physical problems was broadly observed in primitive and ancient cultures (p. 1050). Those who listened to western classical, new age, or Chinese religious music reported significantly lower anxiety and higher levels of satisfaction with their caesarean experiences than the control group did (Tseng et al., 2010). This has resulted in many studies that show the benefit of music to relieve stress and diseases.

While all music has the potential to be therapeutic, music therapy is defined as "the creative and professionally informed use of music in a therapeutic relationship with people identified as needing physical, psychosocial, or spiritual help, or with people aspiring to experience further self-awareness, enabling increased life satisfaction and quality" (Rykov, 2008).

The experience of improvised music making in the music therapy support group was particularly empowering. This provided opportunities for experiencing feelings of control during a time of loss of control inflicted by the disease and subsequent experiences of illness (p. 199).

Several studies have further attested the benefits of music in many areas. A recent study found that music could decrease hyper metabolism by decreasing catecholamine, glucagon, and cortisol. In their investigation, music modified the neuroendocrine-immune axis by increasing growth hormone and decreasing interleukin 6 concentrations. By promoting hypo-metabolism, they concluded that music could act as an additional tool to reestablish metabolic homeostasis in critically ill patients (Nelson & Quick, 1985).

Music therapy has also been shown to have benefits in certain populations, including children. Edwards (2011) asserted that children's cognitive and musical development improved when using music therapy. Another study found that children with autism benefited from music treatments, especially when the music treatments were combined with parental involvement. It was found that music therapy sessions with children who have autism spectrum disorder opens the possibility for positive family outcomes as well as meaningful child development (Thompson, 2012, p. 114; Tseng et al., 2010).

Additionally, the long-term effects of music were studied in groups of preschool children aged 3-4 years who were given keyboard music lessons for six months, during which time they studied pitch intervals, fingering techniques, sight reading, musical notation, and playing from memory. At the end of training, all of the children were able to perform simple melodies by Beethoven and Mozart, which researchers call the Mozart Effect. After they completed the training, they were then subjected to spatial-temporal reasoning tests calibrated for age, and their performance was more than 30% better than that of children of similar ages who were given either computer lessons for 6 months or no special training (Campbell, 2009).

A large area of research shows music has great effects on the brain. According to Thaut et al. (2009), basic and clinical neuroscience research in music and brain function have driven a paradigmatic change in music therapy from a socio-cultural base using interpretative models of music to a neuroscience base using active perception and performance models. The authors stated that neurologic music therapy has established evidence-based therapeutic techniques to retrain and re-educate brain and behavior functions in neurologic disorders and injuries, particularly in the area of motor recovery in stroke (pg. 6).

Neurologic music therapy is defined as the therapeutic application of music to cognitive, affective, sensory, language, and motor dysfunction due to disease or injury to the human nervous system (Thaut et al., 2009, p. 406). Music was found to access control processes in the brain related to control movements, attention, speech production, learning, and memory, which can help retain and recover functions in the injured or disease brain (p. 407). Additionally, neuroscience and music have synergistic effects. Shannon and LaGasse (2013) uncovered two critical findings that transpired from the efforts of neuroscience and music. First, brain areas used during music perception and production are not exclusive to music, and second, music learning changes the brain. These findings have helped to identify the underlying scientific mechanisms for change, growth, and learning that can result from music therapy (p.12).

CHAPTER 7

How Do I Meditate?

"Let the things on earth I borrow create fruits for tomorrow." —Estella Chavous

THERE ARE VARIOUS BELIEFS on how to meditate, but the actual success comes when one puts forth their desire to learn and sets aside a commitment to practice. Regardless of the style chosen, the benefits far outweigh the risks. For those of you who are ready to take on the meditation challenge, here are some suggested considerations to get the process into motion.

The first thing to do is to "GROUND" yourself for successful change. This takes real commitment, so if you're just getting started, you might want to investigate using one of the many change models available. There are different types of change models modeled after Lewin (1947) and Kotter (2002), pioneers of change, and more recently by Dean and Ackerman (2015). All of these change models were developed to prepare individuals so that they can successfully implement change. A platform that we use is The Chavous/Chavous-Kambach

GROUND change model, developed to inspire positive individual change. Its 6 steps prepare you for *Getting acclimated to your environment, Realizing your vision, Opening your mental capacity, Using your inner strength, Noticing wins and conflicts, and Dedicating yourself for effective and continual commitment for change.* The model supports you by suggesting change steps that you document while experiencing your meditative practice. The Chavous/Chavous Kambach GROUND model was specifically designed to help individuals through individual and collective change.

LEARNING TO AVOID DISTRACTIONS

Many of you might be thinking something like "all of this sounds good, but how am I going to realistically avoid distractions?" One woman wrote:

"There is no way that my demanding boss, my addicting cell phone, or my busy, draining lifestyle is going to make room for this practice. Additionally, how do I continue this practice once I start it with the hectic life I lead?

I am a single parent woman who has experienced a really stressful day at work. I start at 7 a.m. and leave work at 3:30 p.m. just in enough time to rush to pick my children up from school. I have to stop and get a few groceries, which leaves me to arrive home at 5 p.m. I fix my kids a quick snack before preparing dinner, and we sit down to eat it at 6:30 p.m.

By the time we're done eating, putting the food away, and doing the dishes it's 7:30. I remember my practice and immediately go into my room at 7:45 to meditate for 10 minutes. But 4 minutes into my meditation, one of my children knocks on the door. I did not get in 10 minutes as planned. What should I do?"

Not getting through a practice or being interrupted is a common occurrence not just for single mothers but for everyone. So what is the best way to deal with distractions that unexpectedly come your way during meditation? Does the mother tell her child she's busy, or does she talk to the child and then resume later? When she does resume, does she have 6 minutes to go, or should she start the whole 10 minutes over again? Should I accept a conference meeting WebEx that just got put on my schedule and delay my meditation until lunch? How can I tell my boss and co-workers that I meditate at a certain time and can't be on the call or in the meeting?

Distractions, whether internal or external or personal or professional, are a part of most meditations. These distractions should be acknowledged and handled based on good judgment at the time. It is important that expectations are set with work and family that let them know that you have allotted this specific time every day for the practice. This may take juggling time slots for a while, but believe me everyone will get the message. During the time that you meditate, it might be a good idea to have an activity planned for your child that you know will keep their attention. If they interrupt, you can ask them to join you in quiet time. During this time (if it works) or with any distraction that took you away from your meditation, gently guide your attention back to your practice. Learning how to manage through the distraction is part of the learning process, but with preparation and set expectations you will command that time for you. Here are tips that can help you.

- Set a time expectation where you are not available, and under most circumstances you should not change this.

- Plan for emergencies or urgent events prior to your time slot.

- Turn off all cell phones, televisions, computers, or anything that beeps.

- Learn to acknowledge the distraction in your mind, letting it leave slowly as you go back to your meditative state.

- If you only get in a limited amount of time and not the full 10 minutes, you still have benefited from the experience.

DEALING WITH A STRESSFUL EPISODE

Stressful episodes are other considerations to work through during meditation. One gentleman shared his experience below, questioning how to handle it.

"John sits down to meditate in his relaxed, high-rise penthouse suite. He has an audio of the sound of wind chimes, and he has set his attention to just relax and focus on the sound of the wind chimes for 10 minutes.

One minute into his 10 minutes of meditation, he cannot shake the anxiety that comes from the disagreement he had with his parents. He begins to mentally replay argument after argument that he has been having with his parents over his wanting to marry the girl he's dated for the last 5 years. He tries to focus back on the wind chimes, but he cannot block out the visuals of his parents screaming at the thought of him bringing her into his family. At this point, he wasn't sure if he should allow his meditation to take place or let this mental interruption win."

John's situation is not unfamiliar. Stressful situations are a constant part of our lives, but how we deal with these trials and tribulations is what is important. The art of meditation is designed to help us manage through these stresses so that we can find that place of calm. By doing this, we are going through what some call a mental healing, taking us to better places of resolve. It takes practice, but continuing through the tough thoughts that come into your head, liked John's, results in the beginning of the healing process. When these stressors surface, acknowledge them, then gently bring your mind back to that sacred word, mantra, prayer, guided voice, chime, breath, or whatever meditation technique you have chosen at the time. This may also be a good time to experiment with different forms of meditation or work with a meditation guide to help with your particular needs.

ENVIRONMENTAL CONCERNS

One factor that we often hear about is that a person's environment is not conducive to meditation. One person wrote:

> "We hear this all the time in our practice. "Should I take breaks in the car . . . go into a room in the library . . . take a walk to the park . . . or close my office or bedroom door?" The answer to those questions is that anywhere safe is a good place to take 10 minutes to meditate. No matter where you are there could be distractions, and you won't be able to create that perfect ambiance at all times. Being able to be in an environment that may seem less than perfect actually increases your practice in that it challenges you to push through the thoughts and distractions to find your place of peace. That is what it is all about, conditioning your mind to get past distractions or events that trouble you. So, if you have that bad day at work that started at 10 am, you should take a break to re-group through your meditative practice as soon as time permits, enabling you to find that special place no matter where you are.

You might also find that you want to go through this meditative experience alone, with a group, or through a combination of both. It is nice to start with a meditation coach or team as it creates a forum so that discussion can be shared regarding your experience. Someone else has experienced many of the things you are experiencing at this early stage, and it helps to talk through these things so that you can break through any barriers preventing you from fully benefiting from the practice. Setting a location or place of calm for you during your meditation is important. Some use candles, oils, incense, and/or labyrinths, all of which create the right setting for your practice. Experiment with this individually and in groups and try to cultivate that experience wherever you practice. Remember that meditation is patience in training. To commit to connect takes patience and persistence. Athletes don't get strong overnight, and it's okay if you don't either. Here are tips for overcoming environmental constraints.

- Decide how long and where you're going to practice.

- Meditation is a special time, so be in the moment no matter where it is.

- Practice in different settings to build self-awareness and reflection.

- Learn and grow from each distraction and experience.

MEDITATIVE TECHNIQUES

One thing that is helpful is the use of differing meditative techniques. These range from sound techniques (mantras), affirmations (focusing on a phrase important to you), music (natural or soothing sounds, bells, chimes, singing bowls, etc.), visualization (personal images, places), and movement (yoga, dance, walking). An example is in the use of personal mantras, which are positive phrases or affirmative statements that you say to yourself for the purpose of motivation or encouragement. This could be your favorite quote, proverb, spiritual truth, or religious saying that motivates and inspires you.

Below are some examples.

"Ask for what you want and be prepared to get it." —*Maya Angelou*

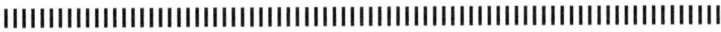

||||||||||||||||||||||||||||||||||||||||||||||||||||||||||||||||||||||||||

"Excellence does not require perfection." —*Henry James*

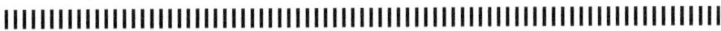

||||||||||||||||||||||||||||||||||||||||||||||||||||||||||||||||||||||||||

"Don't put a question mark where God has put a period." —*Joel Osteen (via Kim)*

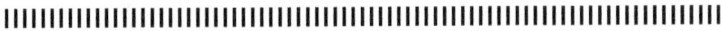

||||||||||||||||||||||||||||||||||||||||||||||||||||||||||||||||||||||||||

SUMMARY

Now that you have gone through the change model, found a good environment and experienced a technique that you like, it is important that you work on body awareness. A good meditation coach can help you with breathing, energy flow, and focus and can help guide you to a relaxing state. There are many ways to access coaches and training in meditation. A good place to start is a yoga center or places or people specializing in holistic training. Once you have found a coach, you will see that the cost varies. Some sessions are free with an add-on to other services. These are nominal in price and often contain a series of trainings that teach a certain type or style. Elite gyms and community centers are now offering meditation, so it is easy to find qualified coaches in your area. Lastly, the Internet, YouTube, podcasts, blogs, and phone apps are great ways to find qualified meditation experts who can take you through a meditation routine that can be done in person or online.

Many have found that they would rather use a guide because it helps them spend their time relaxing and not having to remember to focus on some parts of the practice, but others enjoy the personal time alone. This is the great thing about meditation—it is an experience that is individual and personal.

A goal of meditation is to open one's mind to any occurring thought, sensation, or emotion and consequently expand the consciousness to a place where one reaches clarity. You may not know this, but most people have created this place for themselves. That's why we know the difference between happiness and unhappiness. Through meditation, you can imagine being in that place any time, allowing your body, mind, and soul to have time for you. You will be surprised at the answers to questions, creativity, healing, and clarity all gained from this all-encompassing gift.

CHAPTER 8

Real Life Meditation Stories

"Life to me is love, fun, interactive, and an experience in the stages of one's life."
—Natalia Cota-Kambach (12 years old)

IN THIS SECTION of *Let Meditation Mend You,* we will share with you stories of how meditation has helped resolve some of life's most stressful situations. What better way to understand the benefits of meditation than to hear how different stressors have affected others? It is our hope that you will read these stories knowing that your situation can better be coped with by taking on this practice and that no matter how difficult the situation or goal, the practice of meditation has had profound effects on those who have practiced it.

There are a lot of people who want to meditate but are looking for a guide, technique, or explanation that helps them get started. It is important to note that each of the following individuals realized a positive change with only a few minutes of meditation a day, and they were able to turn their attention off of the flood of anxious thoughts that overwhelmed them to actions that helped them positively address those anxious thoughts.

As you read through these stories, know that we have only picked some of the most common stress factors that plague our society. It is also important to note that even good things or events cause stress, so being prepared for any disruptive change good or bad is what we are aiming for. We are all going to have stress in our lives, but how we respond and control it is what is important.

Juliana's Bullying Story

Bullying has become an epidemic in American society. It is defined as unwanted, aggressive behavior among school aged children involving a real or perceived power imbalance (StopBullying.gov). Countless studies have shown improvements in health-related effects like behavioral conditions through implementing sitting-meditative practices among youth aged 6 to 18 years in school, clinic, and community settings across all meditation modalities, including mindfulness meditation, transcendental meditation, mindfulness-based stress reduction, and mindfulness-based cognitive therapy (Land, 2008). Outreach and awareness campaigns to victims of bullying can increase self-worth and more importantly save lives.

> Juliana was 6 when she was brought to this country from overseas. Her parents immigrated to the U.S. under the worst of conditions. The only English she knew was what she heard on TV or through a passing American who seemed like a foreigner to her. Her Spanish was great and so was her IQ, but due to her inexperience with the English language, she was pushed further and

further behind in school. To complicate things even more, her classmates would do mean things to her— eating her lunch, asking her to give up her chair, taking her belongings, and continuously chanting harsh words and threats. Her parents would console her but would tell her to just work to get along and fit in, not knowing the seriousness of bullying problems in schools.

One day, an unexpected, life-changing event happened. A substitute teacher, Ms. Wells, filled in for her regular teacher. Juliana felt a real connection to her as did the other children, even the troubled ones. On day 2 of her filling in with Juliana's class, she announced that she had gotten approval from the parents and school district to conduct a pilot program that involved the class partici- pating in quiet time for 10 minutes. There wasn't much protest because 10 minutes away from course work is welcomed in most classrooms. The program went on for 3 months, and although Juliana's regular teacher came back, Ms. Wells still conducted the 10-minute sessions throughout the time allotted.

Those three months changed Juliana's life as well as the lives of her bullies. The class didn't notice it at first, but a peaceful calm was among the students and everyone who took part in the quiet time. Everyone seemed less abusive, more tolerant, and less angry. The program pilot was continued well past Ms. Wells' departure with unbelievable results. As for Juliana, she is in high school, an honor student, fluent in English, liked by the students, and a youth who practices meditation daily. If it hadn't been for that experience with Ms. Wells, Juliana questions where she would be today.

Kari's Job Loss Story

A recent survey conducted by CareerBuilder showed that 38% of the workforce is currently managed by a millennial. This generation is predicted to be the largest segment of the workforce. One issue that was found in the study was that young managers show a strong preference for hiring other younger workers. This can leave older workers feeling alienated and squeezed out of the workplace, causing stress and depression. This type of stress is real but, the use of meditation has helped manage it. Choosing like-minded career individuals happens ill-respective of age, race, or any other identifier. Work will have to be done to bring awareness to the issue of employment and older workers. Kari's story sheds light on the issue and how using meditation helped her overcome her misfortune.

Kari spent most of her career in the same business. She was successful and good at what she did. However, she went through a huge shock recently when she was unexpectedly let go for a younger person who had less experience but was more technology savvy. She was humiliated, angry, and hurt at first, but soon afterwards she began to feel the real fear that this loss of a job would throw her into financial turmoil. Depression and increased anxiety began to set in, especially around the uncertainty in her job future and lifestyle change.

A younger former co-worker who continually stayed in contact with her asked her numerous times to attend a group meditation session. Until then she had declined with multiple excuses, but the 10-day rain and cloudy skies in Seattle influenced her to finally give in; she was looking for any way possible to end this slump downward into deeper and deeper depression. It was taking a toll on her, but she forced herself that day to gain enough strength to make it to the community center's meditation class. Feeling disempowered initially, she took part in the experience, which was scary yet intriguing.

The voice guided her to a place of calm that she knew but had forgotten about in the last few months. It was a place that always made her smile and feel that there was not a worry in the world. This was for her a special place in Hawaii that she always reflected on when asked about good memories. After the session, many shared their experiences with the group, and she realized that (1) she was not alone and (2) there was a place in her memory that she could use to escape the mental challenges of life to find calm. She began to meditate 2-5 minutes a day and in 1 month had a new job and newfound passion. She now meditates using a routine of 10 minutes a day with three other members of that same meditation group.

Candice's Moving Story

Moving can be exciting or unpromising, but either way it is very stressful. Many of us are nesters, needing to feel and be assured of the security and safety of our homes. The disruptive change of moving, whether it be caused by good or bad circumstances, can cause ill effects and stress for us all. Candice's story shows how forgetting regular routines (like meditation) during heightened times of stress can be conquered through meditation.

It was 2 weeks before the move date, and Candice had gotten up early to go through her checklist. Packing up all of their belongings and then unpacking them was a hassle, but she was thankful that they had hired someone to do all of this labor for them. Normally, Candice would be off to her normal daily routine of meditation, a long walk or the gym, but today she instead looked at the long, dreaded list before her. As she looked at all the things she had to do to prepare for the move, she started feeling a bit of anxiety. The interesting thing is that she hadn't felt anxiety in months. Her meditation and exercise routine kept her stress free most of the time.

Candice started to try to work through the feeling, but a big sense of fear came over her. "What are we doing? Leaving our friends, family, and routines all for a career opportunity that we really weren't sure of! My husband

and I both wanted to take advantage of the move out of California due to the promotional opportunity and lower cost of living that New Mexico offers. We are renting out our current home, but what if the tenants don't pay or if we can't find jobs that will bring us back!" Beads of sweat began to dampen Candice's forehead, and her heart began to race. She called Eugenia, a friend of hers who is always grounded, to see if she could help calm her down.

Eugenia quickly answered the phone, and she could immediately tell by Candice's voice that she wasn't quite right. Before Candice could talk, Eugenia began to lead her in a guided meditation session on the phone. At that moment, Candice remembered that wonderful release and calm her meditation session brought to her. As she listened to Eugenia guiding her to that place of calm, she lost focus for a bit, beating herself up about not having meditated since the move was announced. "Up until now all was normal without it, but I should have known this could happen" she thought. Then she remembered to do as she had learned in meditative practice, which was to acknowledge the thought and then to release it and take herself back to her breathing.

Her mind drifted to her favorite corner in the room where she would light her sacred candle and incense to begin her practice. It's interesting that she could imagine *all of this with her phone in her ear. Eugenia went on for 10 minutes, and then they sat in silence for 5. As lovely bells rang, taking them out of the deep peace of their meditation, Candice was so thankful for the fellowship and the peace she was given. "What would I do without you, Eugenia?" Candice asked. Eugenia replied, "just like we did today . . . I am only a phone call, Skype, or text away."*

Three months passed and Candice was now in her new home. That day taught her several things: (1) distance does not affect fellowship; (2) you can create your place of calm anywhere, and (3) be disciplined about your meditation practice, even when you're not in a stressful time.

Tony's Cancer Story

Major illnesses are huge stressors in life. This stress can be felt by not only the person sick, but also all those involved in their care. These illnesses can be acute or chronic, and they affect us emotionally. Depression is a very common reaction to sickness, and so is development of negative behavior. In the story below, Tony dealt with the stress by using meditation to get him through his recently diagnosed cancer.

Tony was a very active and fit middle-aged man. He belonged to a very elite fitness club in his area and used that facility as a place to not only workout but also to socialize with his friends. To his friends he was the picture of health. However, after being diagnosed with cancer, he fell out of his fitness routine and hadn't been to the gym in a while. A few weeks before, his friends had really started calling him and insisting on him meeting them. He decided to break the news to them and meet them at the juice bar at the gym.

It was difficult at the bar. Everyone commented that he looked even healthier and fitter even though he hadn't been to the gym. Normally he would boast and tell them they needed to do a few more sets, but today he had to tell them the bad news of his recent diagnosis of prostate cancer. It was very hard for him, especially because he was in their eyes the picture of perfect health. After he broke the news, his friends were shocked, but they started to share their challenges with health not only in their lives but also in the lives of others they've known. This surprised him, and he felt sorry that he hadn't known his friends' struggles earlier.

While in discussion they shared their support for him, and one invited him to a meditation class he was attending later in the day after their meeting. Meditation was "out there" to Tony, but because he had recently read an article about the universal platform that didn't involve religion, he decided to give it a try. At this point, he thought "why not?" and agreed to join him. He entered the class, and the meditation leader explained the *principles of the class as he led them through a guided practice. He also shared a meditation CD and a pamphlet that contained benefits, origins, beliefs, and evolutions of meditation after the class.*

Tony got through the cancer and side effects, and his health got back to where it was before his diagnosis. He has now added a routine that includes daily meditation. The results have been amazing in that he was able to find that place of calm during his stressful time and believes that the stresses in his life if maintained could have prevented his sickness in the first place. He uses meditation regularly because it has added to his total well-being.

Ria's Self-image and Being a Teen Story

If you have any interaction with kids (or if you have gone through puberty yourself), you know how puberty affects teenagers physically and emotionally. They are concerned with not only the perfect body image, but also how they are perceived and fit in with their peers. Ria's story shows how attending a yoga class helped her through some of the experiences she was going through as a teen.

Ria didn't know what happened to her this year, but she woke up one morning not knowing who that other person was she was looking at in the mirror. She had felt so self-confident before, but at this moment she did not like what she saw or felt. She was trying to understand who this person was and get control of her emotional hormones. She felt judged by her friends and misunderstood by her parents. All the pressures to be like the images on the magazines, television, and social media were stressful and she was just feeling out of control.

Sara, one of her friends, attended a yoga class at one of the centers near her home. As with teenagers, they all began to notice the change in her after her 3-month practice. She was calmer, less concerned with what others or her friends thought, and had started to build a unique look for herself. She was more focused and seemed more engaged.

Ria asked if she could attend a few classes with Sara. Ria felt intimidated at first, but then the experience overwhelmed her and created a transformation that she began to love. She was still hormonal and sometimes affected by her peers' thoughts, but she, like Sara, was beginning to transform both in mind and body.

Jennifer's Student Stress Story

Academic problems like poor grades, inability to retain information, problems with teachers, and inability to meet deadlines are common to students of all ages. In addition, stress, anxiety, and depression were all reported as top factors that negatively impact academic performance. In 2012, a National College Health Assessment Report found that within the last 12 months, 55.5% of undergraduate students and 57.1% of graduate students experienced "more than average" or "tremendous amounts of stress". Furthermore, 6.1% of undergraduate and 4.4% of graduate students are seen by a mental healthcare professional at their campus Counseling Services (USC College, National College Health Assessment Report, 2012, p. 5). It was also found that stress could be managed through meditation. Below is Jennifer's story of student stress and how she managed it through transcendental meditation.

Jennifer went to college late in life. She was a wife and a mother of three with one child on the way. This last pregnancy was unexpected, and although it was a blessing, she felt it would result in her needing to take a break from school. The pressures had already started piling up, and she didn't know if she would be able to keep up. Although supportive, her husband still needed to have the household maintained. Because he was the main provider and they had clearly defined roles, he needed her help sustaining things in the household.

The final days of the semester were approaching, and two main assignments were due. These were also group projects, which required even more time. The first conference call with her class established all the "to do's", and the next one would be a run through of all that was required. After the first call she wanted to quit. How was she going to make time for this when she was sick in the morning, taking kids to school, and preparing for the evening meals and activities? As organized as she was, she didn't think she could do it; mornings were when she did her best work. She began to feel herself fall into a panic and became depressed at the thought of what the outcome of all of this could be.

She started flipping through the radio channels and stumbled on an ad for a transcendental meditation class. She had heard how it helped develop more focus and productivity and had worked really well for students, so she quickly called the number and registered for an upcoming class that fortunately started that week. She attended, learned the practice, and immediately began doing it as a daily routine. The results were amazing, and her meditation routine even helped her with her morning sickness, which may be hard to believe. She was able to get through the school session and was ready to take on more. She can't say enough about how transcendental meditation has changed her life.

Keith and Susan's Divorce Story

Divorce is a major stressor in our lives that affects us in more ways than we can possibly think. In addition to the family impact, it can also affect our finances and our mental and emotional well-being. The turmoil in a family can cause chronic damage to relationships and can leave permanent scars. The story below shows the profound impact that a family vacation to a Buddhist retreat had on their lives.

It was inevitably going to happen . . . Keith and I were divorcing. Our arguments and problems had gotten more intense, and even the counselors had succumbed to divorce being a reality and the best thing for us. The

57

sad part was that we were not only husband and wife but also friends who shared 2 wonderful children together. The stain of our marital problems had become so severe that it began affecting the kids, family, and our friends. Even Keith's work was comprised, resulting in fewer sales and diminished commission, which he had consistently brought into the household. We decided to and filed for divorce, and it was finalized in no time due to our both agreeing to a fair and equitable split.

After the split things were not much better. There was this awkwardness in our family that created a space between us. As I looked at the vacation card in my hand, I remember how we had gotten it. Before the divorce, we attended a Buddhist temple with a family friend, and our family won a trip to a meditation retreat that was being given away. We weren't members of any religion, so the experience of attending was actually good for us. But that was then and this in now. Even though it was free and a planned trip, we were at a different place in our family life, which diminished a lot of enthusiasm of attending. However, with much discussion, we agreed that maybe one last trip as a family might be a good thing, so we headed from Colorado up to Washington for this so called family vacation.

The retreat was all-inclusive, and all we had to do was follow the itinerary given to us. The schedule revolved around family programs, but each had an individual focus. They practiced mindfulness meditation several times a day, and we were able to learn techniques that helped hone in on the skill. We participated in prayers that were going out for world peace, and the activities were geared around the ages of our children and how to develop a happy and peaceful mind. We were there for a week and were changed. The distance we had felt from the divorce disappeared. We were able to talk and not fight, and our kids began to communicate with us again. We have since gone every year and are now practicing mindfulness meditation daily. Although we have not remarried, the relationship that we have now as a family is even better than it was before, and Keith's income has tripled. Meditation not only changed my life but also my entire family's lives.

Colin's Workforce/Work-Life Balance Story

Problems at work can affect how we are at home. If we are not happy, these problems can create a river that spills into our personal lives drowning us and those around us. Many problems with work-life balance have to do with us not being able to separate these two very distinct areas of our lives. This is compounded when these problems have to do with the stability of our homes and the lives we have established for ourselves and for our families. Colin, a very successful designer, tells how centering prayer and meditation brought him back to a focus free from worry and re-established that distinct separation between work and home.

Colin was in a company of constant flux. His company had been purchased several times, and he wasn't sure from day-to-day what that meant for him. He was a strong Christian but felt he was losing his personal experience with Christ due to his preoccupied mind. All he could think about and be consumed with was the change in leadership, position, and possibly employment. At lunch with a colleague, he expressed his frustration with his job and with his mentality. He was never good with change, but this company seemed to be playing a game of Russian roulette with his life. It was affecting his work and home life, and he couldn't separate the two. He just wanted to stop for a moment and think clearly again.

James listened intently and suggested that Colin read up on centering prayer. It is a form of meditation and prayer designed to bring a person closer to Christ. James had started going 2 years ago, and it changed his relationship with God and gave him more clarity and focus at work. Colin had noticed the difference in him and so did others, which was reflected by his recent promotion. Colin agreed to go to the centering prayer meeting the following week during their lunch breaks.

On the day he attended, the leader went over what to expect, what to do, and the basic premise of the practice. He and the others began in silence for 20 minutes,

focusing on a sacred word. As he began to work to fo-
cus, tons of thoughts came to his mind. He had been
told that this was normal and as instructed returned his
thoughts to the sacred word. His first experience at cen-
tering prayer was hard, sitting in silence for that long,
but then it became something he longed for. When the
time came for the session to end, he felt he didn't have
enough time.

As a result of his centering prayer experience, his focus
and attitude were changing, and a few of his colleagues
noticed and even mentioned this to him. He sat with
James at lunch and thanked him for the experience, hop-
ing that he would in some way be able to help share this
experience with others. No longer did he worry about
tomorrow, but he became more thankful each day.

Michelle's Death in the Family Story

Death is part of life, but the death of a loved one is something that causes significant stress. We grieve for our loved ones, and our lives can become permanently seriously disrupted. Michelle tells a story of how meditation helped her deal with the loss of her mother.

I was driving home one night, crying my eyes out. I had
been so not myself, and the cold dreary day in Indiana
didn't help. I realize that death is a part of life, but I
wanted to do so many things with my mom that I wasn't
able to do. It had started to snow and the snow began to

stick to the trees, which meant the expected snowstorm was here. I was minutes away from home, which I was thankful for. It looked like tomorrow would be a snow day, which was nice for me since I was so sad and heavy with grief. I pulled into the garage and went inside. In the mirror I saw how bad I looked. I kept thinking that I hoped I didn't look this bad in front of my peers and co-workers and that it was no wonder people seemed to be avoiding me.

My home was my castle and everything was beautiful just like I had worked so hard to create, but even that didn't help. I would give it all up just for one more day with my mom. I turned on and off the radio, hating the music, and went into the kitchen to look at my mail. In the stack was a flash drive from "The Guided Meditation Experts" that asked me to try this free introductory session.

I went to my computer and opened up the drive to listen. It had the most calming nature sounds, and the woman's voice was so relaxing. She took me to places in the woods that really connected me to my mom, who loved going hiking with me. I at one point felt that she was walking right alongside of me as we watched the owl in the highest tree limb and the deer grazing in the grass. I imagined seeing her jump when the brush started moving, laughing when it was just a group of *rabbits running for protection from something bigger than them.*

When the session ended, I felt like I had not only experienced meditation but also time with my mom. I slept like a baby and for the first time actually had a dream that I remember! I enrolled to get several of their CDs and downloaded them and now listen to them religiously every night. I will say that there is not a day that I don't miss my mom, but the visualization and messages that I am getting from the meditation let me know that she is with me all the time.

Taryn's Weight-loss Story

The truth to weight is that everyone has beauty no matter his or her size. At times influences from magazines, media, health concerns, or simple goals of looking a certain way can cause the desire for one to begin a program to lose weight. The journey to weight loss is one that takes dedication, determination, and persistence. Taryn's story highlights how her journey led to success with the use of music and meditation. She used 5-10 minutes of meditation with a focus on words that ignited an amazing change in her life.

Taryn had always struggled with being comfortable in her own skin. She was overweight and was having a difficult time getting the energy to make the change to a healthier lifestyle for years. One thing Taryn did love was nature. Her love for nature inspired creativity, inspired her to take pictures, and also inspired an occasional walk on a nearby trail.

One beautiful day in September, Taryn decided it would be great to go by the nearby trail to take pictures. When she got on the trail, she saw three rabbits next to each other and began taking pictures. She looked for a better angle when she noticed the fourth eating and noticeably heavier than the rest. She looked at the heavier rabbit and thought of herself. It was time for the change.

She remembered her sister saying how she used meditation and music to aid in a healthier lifestyle and thought she would try the same. Every day, Taryn decided to go to the trail and walk for 30 minutes, stop and take pictures, and then meditate with the use of music for 10 minutes. By the end of the month, Taryn had lost 13 lbs. and had the motivation to up her game on exercise and getting to a better self.

Kara's Dating Story

A relationship of any kind takes work. At their best relationships can bring joy and contentment, but at their worst they can cause stress and pain. The story of Kara tells how meditation can aid in the healing process. Kara used meditation to soothe and conquer her pain that resulted from an unsuccessful relationship.

Kara was in a relationship where manipulation and anger were its primary components. Her relationship ended abruptly, and soon after she began to feel worn down and stressed because she missed the relationship. Kara loved animals and usually found peace with them. She was distraught after the break up and decided to try and redirect herself by meditation with a focus on animals that she loved.

Every day got easier, but she still longed to call her ex on a regular basis. Every time she thought of calling, she would take 2 to 5 minutes to close her eyes and meditate. She would start by thinking of her little pup "Tiger" who was in her eyes her power animal. Then she would focus on the word heal. Sometimes she would cry when the thoughts and words would enter her mind, but it was all part of the healing process and she was able to not make a phone call or text.

After 10 days she was feeling that she had more control and was able to get her life on track. By 15 days, she felt she was able to enjoy things with friends without thinking of her ex too often, and she was able to now ignore his calls. By 30 days, she was feeling like she did before she met him. Allowing time to mourn the relationship and heal with meditation was key to her process.

CHAPTER 9

Grounding Yourself for a Successful Meditative Practice

LEARNING TO GROUND YOURSELF FOR SUCCESS

There are many approaches to a successful meditative practice but it starts with grounding yourself. The *Chavous/Chavous-Kambach Ground Change Guide* consists that can help you have a better practice. These six steps prepare you to *Get acclimated to your environment, Realize your vision, Open your mental capacity, Use your inner strength, Notice and be aware of the wins and conflicts, and Dedicate yourself for effective and continual renewal.* This change model starts with the foundation of awareness, realization, and openness then continues on to use, noticing, and dedication. In any meditation practice grounding yourself will help you reach your desired state of calm and give you a more focused intention for the practice.

G et acclimated to your environment

R ealize your vision

O pen your mental capacity

U se your inner strength to make change

N otice and be aware of the wins and conflicts

D edicate yourself for effective and continual change

Get acclimated to your environment

- A successful practice involves not only preparing but also acclimating yourself to the environment. It involves the process of adjusting oneself into it gradually no matter what condition or distraction presents itself. Meditation can be practiced in all types of environments; it just takes creating your personal space in spite of any circumstance. The key is not letting the environment limit you or the practice.

Realize your vision

- This is accomplished by establishing a vision that is a place of calm for you. This vision needs to be real and personal. You should be engaging in and connected to this place so much that your senses respond to it. Realization can be accomplished through affirmations, spot checks, and reminders that support it.

Open your mental capacity

- Open your mental capacity through meditation. It helps you form the habit of becoming more focused and less worried about discomfort. You become more appreciative of the thing's life offers you and, in the process, start to develop a better understand of how to control the clutter in your mind. Your meditative practice helps you form habits and opens you up to awareness, choices, and freedom.

Use your inner strength to make change

- Although inner strength comes from within, we sometimes don't realize the power of our strength until we dig deep into ourselves. There are specific traits and concepts that typically make up inner strength but the acknowledgment of these is in our acceptance that all seasons in life are meaningful. We must learn to draw from our strengths in these seasons and the practice of meditation helps us do this.

Notice the small and big wins and what prevents your vision

- Notice and be aware of wins and conflicts in your meditation practice. Life should not be taken for granted nor should one give into the conflict. Extend well wishes that includes compassion, kindness, appreciation, honoring cherishing, and love. Celebrate your life and the life of others.

Dedicate yourself for effective and continual change

- Renewal is the act of being made new, fresh, or strong again and this is accomplished by being completely entrenched in your meditative practice. It takes setting an enthusiastic agreement with yourself. If meditation is practiced regularly and you have dedicated yourself to it, the renewal process will be automatic and sustainable.

CHAPTER 10

The *Let Meditation Mend You* GROUNDING Guide

PUTTING THE GROUNDING GUIDE INTO PRACTICE

Get Acclimated—Some of the major environmental factors are influenced by time, place, space, climate and noise. Before you begin your meditation practice, work to identify potential factors that might come into play before your practice begins. Try to remove the ones in your control like the closing of a window, shutting of a door, or silencing a cell phone. For those you can't control work to acknowledging them in your practice. After you have acknowledged them begin to release them out of your thoughts by returning to your mantra, scripture, affirmation, breathing, or whatever focus you have set.

Guide Tips:

- **Remember meditation is not a judgmental practice.** Only concern yourself with awareness of the environment, but not with it being a pitfall to a successful practice.

- **Most of what we recall during a meditation practice is a recent thought.** Processing current thoughts is a normal process. A good best practice is to go over and bring awareness to this before the practice so you can move freely into a practice state.

- **Stay attentive to the practice and remind yourself that you are meditating.** When a distractive moment occurs, it is normal to get sidetracked. Don't let it stop you from enjoying the moment but rather began to re-focus binging yourself back to the present.

- **Refocus the problems that occur in your practice.** It is up to you to bring the correct re-focusing back to your practice. If it is a posture problem re-adjust; if you are in pain engage in diaphragmatic (deep) breathing speaking to yourself in positive acceptance. This can be difficult depending on the situation, but controlling the moment takes time. Do things only to the best of your ability.

Contemplation:

How will you acclimate to your meditative practice?

_____

_____

_____

Realize your Vision—Most individuals do not visualize where they want their practice to take them. Nothing is wrong with this as the main goal of meditations is to go beyond the mind to find an area of happiness and bliss. If the mind and all of its clutter is an obstacle to finding your bliss, the ritual of setting intentions and visions can enhance the practice helping you manifest the things you want and feel, helping you process and create it.

Guide Tips:

- **Be specific in your vision or intention.** The best way to give your intention or vision value is to be specific. This specificity should embrace your dreams and goals giving them real power.

- **Manifest what your vision looks like.** A vision defines your optimal desired state in the future state. It tells you what to achieve and gives you the why. Work to define your dreams so they manifest both internally and externally.

- **Develop affirmations that support it.** Choose an affirmation that works for you. Remember that conscious thoughts are what supports you. Your vision or affirmation should focus on you having what you want and how it looks in the present moment.

- **Have a spirit of gratitude.** Consistent gratitude will amplify your life, focus, and your vision will flourish. Get out of your old mindset and walk in a new mindful presence.

Contemplation:

How will you use meditation to manifest your vision?

_____

_____

_____

Open your mental capacity—When your mind is thriving so do too. It has been shown that meditation preserves the brains gray matter, slowing down the rate of gray matter loss which is the cause of stress and bad health. We can support this by ensuring that we pay attention to our brain health and open ourselves up to slowing down the failing neurons that cause bad health.

Guide Tips:

- **Develop a routine and habit for brain health.** Forming a habit of a daily meditative practice improves total wellbeing.

It relieves anxiety and depression and improves attention and concentration. Establish this habit for overall psychological wellbeing.

- **Perform a daily check in with yourself.** The opening of your mind takes performing daily check ins with yourself. This is not only a best practice but making this a regular routine trains the mind to take notice. Before you dive into anything take a few moments to check in with yourself and others.

- **Heart centered practices involved quieting the mind.** A skill we are rarely taught is listening. Meditation allows us time to quiet our minds enabling us to listen to all aspects of our being. Allow yourself to experience the mental, physical, and spiritual aspects in being still.

- **Get to know yourself through learning and training.** The practice of meditation isn't just about focusing or emptying your mind. It's about learning how your mind works, learning what's in and should be in it, and ultimately putting the right things in their right place. That's when the true healing starts and the learning process begins.

Contemplation:

How will you be still and perform daily check in to uncover your feeling?

_____

_____

_____

Use Meditation to increase your inner strength—You possess the innate inner strength to create a powerful meditative practice. Model and live this transformation as it will be visible in all you do. Acknowledge the change in yourself when noticed by others and let it guide you along the way. Use your meditative practice for continual growth and development within yourself and for the support of others.

Guide Tips:

- **Acknowledge your change for continued growth.** This requires you to use the capacity required to recognize something about the new you. You then must own it and celebrate the groundbreaking change it has made within you.

- **Model the behavior and be aware of how it affects others.** As you become aware of your inner strength use it to model behavior for others. Replace stress for calm and weakness for strength. Be quick to hear, slow to speak and slow to anger.

- **Give rise to the Atmabala—*the strength of the soul.*** Your inner strength is your core and the strength of the soul comes through faith and obedience.

- **Become your own best friend.** Enjoy spending time with yourself and watching the noticeable progress you make. The breakthroughs come from emotional intelligence. Like what to see yourself and congratulate yourself often.

Contemplation:

How will you use the inner strength found through meditation to support life seasons?

_____

_____

_____

Notice be aware of wins and conflicts—Understand your stressors and what prevents you from reaching that place of calm. Regardless of the source, take time to remove it from your life or control the effects it has on you. After you incorporate this into your daily routine, you will be better able to calm yourself when faced with any challenge.

Guide Tips:

- **Utilize Body scans in your practice.** An important part of any meditative practice is the use of body scans to bring awareness to wholeness. It helps with your thoughts, emotions, and physical sensations resulting in heightened awareness and confidence.

- **Start you day don't let it start you.** Starting your day is a great way to set a positive routine for the day. It helps to support a good day and helps to overcome challenges should it not go so well. Although you may experience a challenge that is hard to overcome, using this routine daily will ensure a good day the majority of the time.

- **Understand your stressors.** We all have a breaking point and can be thrown into fight or flight for different reasons. The key is to know what triggers spin you into a stressful state and work on ways to counteract it.

- **Face conflict.** It is hard for many people to handle conflict. In the Kilmann conflict resolution theory, avoiding, compromising, accommodating and collaborating are strategies that can be used to overcome it. Mediation can be used in conflict resolution as conflict starts from within. Meditation helps one approach a change in behavior creating a positive outcome for everyone.

Contemplation:

How will you celebrating wins and overcome conflict?

_____

_____

_____

Dedicate yourself for effective and continual renewal—Change is good and renewal is too! It takes consistency to see continual results in a meditation practice. This means getting into a daily meditation routine and making this a priority in your life.

Guide Tips:

- **Establish a meditation routine.** Studies have shown that meditating for only 10 minutes a day is all you need to experience positive benefits. Set a daily routine so you will experience continued success.

- **Assess and reassess your goals and vision.** Vision and goals change. One of the values of meditation can be seen in how well one navigates through these changes maintaining clarity and focus. Meditation is proven to be a successful tool in emotional intelligence and sustaining positive change.

- **Continue to implement and act on areas of difficulty.** Meditations help to improve the mind, body, and heart. It has a relaxation response that helps in all areas of wellbeing. With that said, each person has an area of their life that is personally challenging. It is important to address this area with more effort, focus, and support. This can be with meditation or with other traditional and non-traditional practices.

Pay it forward to others— This is the act of asking a person to repay your kindness by doing a good deed for someone else. This helps you earn trust and inspires generosity and compassion. It helps us with the dedication and renewal area as we began focusing on the broader concept of kindness for ourselves and others.

Contemplation:

How will you sustain the renewal process?

_____

_____

_____

The *Let Meditation Mend You* GROUND guide is intended to help you prepare and experience a greater meditative practice. Once you establish yourself in a daily practice these tips will become natural process. A good best practice is for you to journal your experiences. These can later be used as a reference guide to show you where you begin and where you are going in the mindful meditation transformational journey.

Continued Research

expand our field of research and understand how the GROUND change guide has worked in your lives. Our research will involve us formulating a book with real world experiences on those that have used the Chavous/Chavous-Kambach GROUND Guide. If you are interested in being in the book, please jot down your experiences and send them to us. Take your journal and title it "Grounding for Meditation My Experience". Send it along with your state or country listed in the subject line to us at: *write2@strategicladies.com*.

Looking to get started in meditation?
Strategic Ladies can help. . . .

Strategic Ladies wants their readers to know that they are here to support them with any additional information, research, and practical application of meditation. We can provide information on our program offerings as well as information on additional meditative practices and resources that are available. Our wide variety of services includes workshops, speaker events, consulting, and research.

We can be reached at:

Website: *www.strategicladies.com*

Email: *write2@strategicladies.com*

References

Adams, R. B., & Kirchmaier, T. (2013). Making it to the top: From female labor force participation to boardroom gender diversity. *ECGI-Finance Working Paper,* (347).

Bae, M.J. (2012). *Effect of group music therapy on student music therapists' anxiety, mood, job engagement and self-efficacy.* (72), ProQuest Information & Learning, US. Retrieved from http://libproxy.chapman.edu/login?url=http://search.ebscohost.com/login.aspx?direct=true&AuthType=ip,uid&db=psyh&AN=2012-99050-288&site=eds-live. Available from EBSCOhost psyh database.

Bedford, F. L. (2012). A perception theory in mind-body medicine: guided imagery and mindful meditation as cross-modal adaptation. *Psychonomic Bulletin & Review, 19*(1), 24-45.

Bruscia, K.E. (1989). Defining music therapy. Gilsum, NH: Barcelona.

Buddhist Art—https://en.wikipedia.org/wiki/Buddhist_art

Douglas M. Burns *Buddhist Meditation and Depth Psychology.* Access to Insight (Legacy Edition), 30

November 2013, http://www.accesstoninsight.org/lib/authors/wheel088.html.

Burns, D. M. (1994). Buddhist meditation and depth psychology.

Campbell, D. (2009). *The Mozart Effect.* New York, NY: HarperCollins.

Campbell, D., & Doman, A. (2011). *Healing at the speed of sound deluxe: how what we hear transforms our brains and our lives.* Retrieved from Penguin.com.

Clair, A. A., & Memmott, J. (2008). *Therapeutic uses of music with older adults.* 2nd ed. Silver Spring, MD: American Music Therapy Association.

Contemplative Outreach—http://www.contemplativeoutreach.org/programs

Csabai, M. (2013). Victorious living-NLP, meditations, affirmations and binaural beats. https://plus.google.com/+MarkCsabai/posts/YrCzbVMsqbA

Davidson, R. J., & McEwen, B. S. (2012). Social influences on neuroplasticity: stress and interventions to promote well-being. *Nature Neuroscience, 15*(5), 689-695.

Department of Labor, W. D. C. B. o. L. S. W. D. C. (2005).

De Vol, T. I. (1974). Ecstatic pentecostal prayer and meditation. *Journal of religion and health, 13*(4), 285-288.

Ding, X., Tang, Y. Y., Tang, R., & Posner, M. I. (2014). Improving creativity performance by short-term meditation. *Behavioral and Brain Functions, 10*(1), 9.

Does cryptic gluten sensitivity play a part in neurological illness? *The Lancet,* Volume 347, Issue 8998, Pages 369—371, 10 February 1996

Doherty, S. E. (2014). *Women Struggle to Reach the Top: Gender Disparities in the Workplace* (Honors Thesis). Retrieved from http://digitalcommons.hamline.edu

Dritsas, A, Platis, C, & Cokkinos, D.V. (2000). Music in a cardiac hospital: clinical application of a brain-heart interaction. *Proceedings of the International Conference of the Onassis Surgery Center;* Dec 7-9; Athens, Greece.

Edwards, J. (Ed.). (2011). *Music therapy and parent-infant bonding.* New York, NY: Oxford University Press

Eisenbarth, C. (2012). Coping profiles and psychological distress: A cluster analysis. *North American Journal of Psychology,* 14(3), 1-6.

Elwér, S., Harryson, L., Bolin, M., & Hammarström, A. (2013). Patterns of gender equality at workplaces and psychological distress. *PloS one, 8*(1), e53246.

Empowering the third billion: women and the world of work in 2012. (n.d).

Fan, Y., Tang, Y., & Posner, M. I. (2014). Cortisol level modulated by integrative meditation in a dose-dependent fashion. *Stress & Health: Journal Of The International Society For The Investigation Of Stress, 30*(1), 65-70.th

Firdaus, S. D., William, B. M., Eric, N., & Bruce, S. M. (2012). Stress-induced redistribution of immune cells—from barracks to boulevards to battlefields: A tale of three hormones—Curt Richter Award Winner. *Psychoneuroendocrinology, 37,* 1345-1368. doi: 10.1016/j.psyneuen.2012.05.008

Grafton, E., Gillespie, B., & Henderson, S. (2010). Resilience: the power within. *Oncology Nursing Forum, 37*(6), 698–705.

Gyamfi, P., Brooks-Gunn, J., & Jackson, A. P. (2001). Associations between employment and financial and parental stress in low-income single black mothers. *Women & Health 2001;32*(1-2):119-35. Taylor & Francis

Hart, R., Ivtzan, I., & Hart, D. (2013). Mind the gap in mindfulness research: A comparative account of the leading schools of thought. *Review Of General Psychology, 17(4),* 453-466. doi:10.1037/a0035212

Hasminda-Hassan, H., Murat, Z.H., Ross, V., Mohd-Zain, Z., & Buniyamin, N. (2011). *Enhancing learning using music to achieve a balanced brain. Engineering Education (ICEED), 2011 3rd International Congress on.* IEEE.

Hawkins, M. (2013). *Mindfulness practices for today's leaders: Reducing stress and improving heart health.* (73), ProQuest Information & Learning, US. Retrieved from http://libproxy.chapman.edu/login?url=http://search.ebscohost.com/login.aspx?direct=true&AuthType=ip,uid&db=psyh&AN=2013-99100-223&site=eds-live Available from EBSCOhost psyh database.

Healthy Heart Meditation—healthy-heart meditation.com

Hill, E., Jacobs, J.L, Shannon, L.L., Brennan, R.T., Blanchard, V.L., & Martinengo, G. (2008). Exploring the relationship of workplace flexibility, gender, and life stage to family-to-work conflict, and stress and burnout. *Community, Work & Family, 11*(2), 165-181.doi:10.100/13668800802027564.

Hindu Meditation—project-Meditaton.org http://www.project-meditation.org/a_mt2/hindu_meditation.html

History of Meditation—Project Meditation –org, by Mary Jones. http://www.projectmeditation.org/wim/history_of_meditation.html

Hölzel, B. K., Lazar, S. W., Gard, T., Schuman-Olivier, Z., Vago, D. R., & Ott, U. (2011). How does mindfulness meditation work? Proposing mechanisms of action from a conceptual and neural perspective. *Perspectives on Psychological Science, 6*(6), 537-559.

Hypnosis definition. American Society of Clinical Hypnosis. Retrieved from http://www.asch.net/public/generalinfoonhypnosis/definitionofhypnosis.aspx

Inflammation. Merriam-Webster's collegiate dictionary, Springfield, Mass.: Merriam-Webster, C2000., 2000. ISBN: 087797080.

John Piper (@JohnPiper)—desiringGod.org

Johnson, H. (2007, June). 'Happy Diwali!' Performance, Multicultural Soundscapes and Intervention in Aotearoa/New Zealand. *In Ethnomusicology Forum* (Vol. 16, No. 1, pp. 71-94). Taylor & Francis Group.

Kaliman, P., Alvarez-Lopez, M. J., Cosín-Tomás, M., Rosenkranz, M. A., Lutz, A., & Davidson, R. J. (2014). Decreased expression of pro-inflammatory genes (RIPK2 and COX2). *Psychoneuroendocrinology, 40,* 96-107.

Kerr, C. E., Sacchet, M. D., Lazar, S. W., Moore, C. I., & Jones, S. R. (2013). Mindfulness starts with the body: somatosensory attention and top-down modulation of cortical alpha rhythms in mindfulness meditation. *Frontiers in human neuroscience, 7.*

Lai, H.L., & Li, Y.M. (2011). The effect of music on biochemical markers and self-perceived stress among first-line nurses: a randomized controlled crossover trial. *Journal of advanced nursing,* 67.11: 2414-2424.

Land, D. (2008). Study shows compassion meditation changes the brain. *University of Wisconsin News.* kansas-city-yoga. com. Published March 25 in the Public Library of Science One.

Madan, S. (2013). The business imperative of gender inclusivity: barriers and bridges. *In Proceedings of International Conference on Business Management & IS* (Vol. 2, No. 1).

Mahmoud, J. S. R., Staten, R. T., Hall, L. A., & Lennie, T. A. (2012). The relationship among young adult college students' depression, anxiety, stress, demographics, life satisfaction, and coping styles. *Issues in mental health nursing, 33*(3), 149-156.

Mason, P. (2014). *Introduction to the lifestory and teaching of Guru Dev Shankaracharya Swami Brahamananda Aaraswati.* Retrieved from http://www. paulmason.info/gurudev/introduction.htmp.

McCreary, S. L., & Alderson, K. G. (2013). The perceived effects of practicing meditation on women's sexual and relational lives. *Sexual and Relationship Therapy, 28*(1-2), 105-119.

McDermott, O., Crellin, N., Ridder, H. M., & Orrell, M. (2013). Music therapy in dementia: a narrative synthesis systematic review. *International journal of geriatric psychiatry, 28*(8), 781-794.

McEwen, B. S. (2013). The brain on stress: toward an integrative approach to brain, body, and behavior. *Perspectives on Psychological Science, 8*(6), 673-675.

McMahon, L. (2013). *Forget the war on women; let's declare a war for women!* (Vol. 79, pp. 357-359): McMurry Inc.

Morgan, N., Irwin, M. R., Chung, M., & Wang, C. (2014). The effects of mind-body therapies on the immune system: meta-analysis. *PloS one, 9*(7), e100903.

Murphy, M. (2002). *The physical and psychological effects of meditation : a review of contemporary meditation research with a comprehensive bibliography. 2nd ed. Annotated update:* Petaluma, CA: Institute of Noetic Science.

Nair, P., & Xavier, M. (2012). Initiating employee assistance program (EAP) for a corporate: an experiential learning. *IUP Journal of Organizational Behavior, 1 1*(2), 67-76.

Nelson, D. L., & Quick, J. C. (1985). Professional women: are distress and disease inevitable? *Academy Of Management Review, 1 0*(2), 206-218. doi:10.5465/AMR.1985.4277941

Nielsen, M. B., & Knardahl, S. (2014). Coping strategies: A prospective study of patterns, stability, and relationships with psychological distress. *Scandinavian Journal Of Psychology, 55*(2), 142-150. doi:10.1111/sjop.12103

Range of Neurologic Disorders in Patients with Celiac Disease: PEDIATRICS Vol. 113 No. 6 June 1, 2004. Immune response to dietary proteins, gliadin and cerebellar peptides in children with autism. *Nutritional Neuroscience 7*(3):151-161, June 2004.

Richardson, P. (2010). There are (still) extra challenges for women business owners. *Inside Tucson Business, 20*(25), 16.

Robb, S.L., Nichols, R.L., Butan, B.L., & Bishop, J.C. (1995). The effects of music assisted relaxation on preoperative anxiety. *Journal of Music Therapy 32*(1), 2-21

Rogers, R. E., & Li, E. Y. (1994). Perceptions of organizational stress among female executives in the U.S. government: An. *Public Personnel Management, 23*(4), 593.

Romano, S. D. (2014). *Leading at the edge of uncertainty: an exploration of the effect of contemplative practice on organizational leaders* (Doctoral dissertation, Antioch University).

Rykov, M. H. (2008). Experiencing music therapy cancer support. *Journal of health psychology, 13*(2), 190-200.

Shannon, K., & LaGasse, A. B. (2013). Music therapy and neuroscience from parallel histories to converging pathways. *Music Therapy Perspectives, 31*(1), 6-14.

Steptoe, A., & Kivimäki, M. (2013). Stress and cardiovascular disease: an update on current knowledge. *Annual review of public health, 34,* 337-354.

StopBullying—gov www.stopbullying.gov/what-is-bullying/definition

Styhre, A. (2013). Sound, silence, music: organizing audible work settings. *Culture & Organization, 19*(1), 22-41. doi: 10.1080/14759551.2011.634197

Tanner, M. A., Travis, F., Gaylord-King, C., Haaga, D. A. F., Grosswald, S., & Schneider, R. H. (2009). The effects of the transcendental meditation program on mindfulness. *Journal of Clinical Psychology, 65*(6), 574-589. doi: 10.1002/jclp.20544 the origin of mindfulness meditation

Teper, R., & Inzlicht, M. (2013). Meditation, mindfulness and executive control: the importance of emotional acceptance and brain-based performance monitoring. *Social cognitive and affective neuroscience, 8*(1), 85-92.

Thaut, M. H., Gardiner, J. C., Holmberg, D., Horwitz, J., Kent, L., Andrews, G., ... & McIntosh, G. R. (2009). Neurologic music therapy improves executive function and emotional adjustment in traumatic brain injury rehabilitation. *Annals of the New York Academy of Sciences, 1169*(1), 406-416.

The New Scofield Reference Bible authorized King James Version

Thompson, G. (2012). Family-centered music therapy in the home environment: promoting interpersonal engagement between children with autism spectrum disorder and their parents. *Music Therapy Perspectives, 30*(2), 109-116.

Thompson, S., & O'Callaghan, C. (2013). Decision making in music therapy: The use of a decision tree. *Australian Journal of Music Therapy, 24,* 48.

Tseng, Y., Chen, C., & Lee, C. S. (2010). Effects of listening to music on postpartum stress and anxiety levels. *Journal of Clinical Nursing, 19*(7-8), 1049-1055. doi: 10.1111/j.1365-2702.2009.02998.x

U.S. Bureau of Labor Statistics, U.S. Department of Labor. *Women in the Labor Force Databook: A Datebook. 2012.* http://www.bls.gov/cps/wlf-databook-2012.pdf. http://www.bls.gov/cps/wlf-databook2007.htm

Vanithamani, M. R., & Menon, S. (2012). Enhancing entrepreneurial success of self-help group (SHG) women entrepreneurs through effective training. *Excel International Journal Of Multidisciplinary Management* zenithresearch.org.in ABSTRACT

Werneburg, B. L., Herman, L. L., Preston, H. R., Rausch, S. M., Warren, B. A., Olsen, K. D., & Clark, M. M. (2011). Effectiveness of a multidisciplinary worksite stress reduction programme for women. *Stress & Health: Journal of the International Society for the Investigation of Stress, 27*(5), 356-364. doi: 10.1002/smi.1380

Wilhoit, J. C. (2014). Contemplative and centering prayer. *Journal Of Spiritual Formation & Soul Care, 7*(1), 107-117.

Will, U., & Berg, E. (2007). Brain wave synchronization and entrainment to periodic acoustic stimuli. *Neuroscience letters,* 424.1 (2007): 55-60.

Yehuda, N. (2011). Music and stress. *Journal of Adult Development, 18*(2), 85-94. doi: 10.1007/s10804-010-9117-4

About the Authors

DRS. ESTELLA & JACINTA CK A.K.A. "Strategic Ladies" work to strategically transform lives. They use bio-individuality approaches, leading to successful and sustainable outcomes. This mother and daughter team founded *Strategic Ladies* based on the need to create actionable and sustainable transformation. They both have lengthy backgrounds in fortune 500 companies whose spectrums range from ground level to leadership positions. This means that they speak your language at all levels. Seeing firsthand the lack of preparedness for stress management especially with women in the workforce led them to team up to create a mission that would raise awareness to alternative treatments like meditation to manage stress.

Together they pursued their doctorate degrees so that they could combine sound research and practical knowledge to their work, resulting in successful outcomes. Their motto of *"We are educated in theory but are practitioners of change"* has resulted in the development of collaborative resources and tools to combat stress using the art of meditation. Their new book *Let Meditation Mend You* introduces you to the various platforms of meditation with a special chapter dedicated to their research with women and stress in the workforce.

You're looking at a woman ...

- You're looking at a woman who was pregnant with her first child and in the midst of a divorce due to her husband's infidelities

- You're looking at a woman who was forced to move in with her parents to make ends meet due to lack of funds and no child support

- You're looking at a woman who had just finished college only to enter a workforce with limited opportunities due to the economic recession

- You're looking at a woman who felt the guilt of bringing a child in the world as she was not prepared at all for the financial responsibility

- You're looking at a woman who was so full of acne scars from stress that people mistook the scars for chicken pox

- You're looking at a woman who felt inferior and because of this was beginning to develop inferior relationships

- You're looking at a woman who was beginning to doubt herself and her self-worth

- You're looking at a woman who moved her way up the corporate ladder only to face real world corporate issues concerning diversity, the "boys' clubs", gender issues, and women not wanting to pay it forward for other women

- You're looking at a woman who worked two jobs to have it all only to fall short of being present, and in the moment, for those who truly mattered

- You're looking at a woman who was visiting every doctor possible until one sat her down warning her that high blood pressure and a-systematic complaints could lead to health and mental concerns

- You're looking at Dr. Stella, a woman who was so full of faith and was losing it to all the stressors in her life

But then something happened. A change in attitude. A miracle. But this miracle wasn't the lottery, or an angel giver, or a knight in shining armor. It turns out that this gift was much, much more. It was the gift of the fight, the survivor, the never give up, the faith that was instilled in me as a child. I then realized that these struggles were causing me to forget my values and my faith. It was then that I open my eyes and began to rise above the struggles.

- I began to pray, meditate, and exercise again

- I began to take time out for me and the ones I love

- I began to appreciate my struggle, my blessing, my daughter, and the fact that I was better than any two-parent home.

- I began to live my purpose and the life that God had for me.

- I began to rekindle prayer and meditation and share it with others, knowing firsthand how it can conquer life struggles

—Dr. Estella

I am ...

I am a woman who was raised by her mom, grandparents, and aunt but never felt deprived

- I am a woman who had trust issues due to my absence of a biological father

- I am a woman who had a well-planned life only to learn that things don't always go as planned

- I am a woman who went through an abusive relationship, hiding them to protect the strength I eluded on the outside

- I am a woman who got married at a very young age not knowing myself well enough to prepare for the responsibility

- I am a woman who was a single mother and although supported by the strength of a great family, felt this life card was an embarrassment

- I am a woman who was accepted to a top law school, which had to be put on hold due to an unplanned pregnancy

- I am a woman that stayed in the forefront of jealously, especially from women who never learned to support each other or how to pay it forward

- I am a woman that finished her masters while with a young child, and starting her doctorate two weeks after her third living child was born

- I am a woman who had her child die in her arms, not realizing that this was even possible

- I am a woman who held her loving grandmother as she passed over to the eternal side

- I am a woman gifted with the gift of discernment, giving prophetic word as God allows

- I am a woman who has developed and improved herself, even through adversity and mistakes along the way

- I am a woman that who is strong in her beliefs and gives all praise and honor to God

- I am woman who loves her friends, family, and those less fortunate

- I am Jacinta a woman that believes life can be stressful, but it is the self-awareness and self-reflection that changes you

This is just a small part of my evolution and experiences that have made me. Every day is a learning experience and with time all wounds heal. A great part of the healing process has been the prayer and meditation that I use in my life. Meditation has helped me frame my purpose and the purpose that God has for me. As my Aunt (Rose), Mom (Estella) and Grammee (Bettie) would say, "Trust in the Lord, turn it over to Him, and meditate on his Word." These words have always resonated with me, but it wasn't until I put them into practice did I see their true benefits.

—Dr. Jacinta CK